MW01533221

VAIL

METHOD

THE
VAIL
METHOD

DR. EHRLICH'S GETTING BETTER NOT JUST OLDER
GUIDE TO

MATTHEW EHRLICH, MD

Copyright © 2020 by Matthew Ehrlich, MD.

All rights reserved. No part of this book may be reproduced or transmitted in any form or by any means, electronic or mechanical, including photocopying, recording, or by any information storage and retrieval system, except in the case of brief quotations embodied in critical articles and reviews, without prior written permission of the publisher.

Although the author and publisher have made every effort to ensure the accuracy and completeness of information contained in this book, we assume no responsibility for errors, inaccuracies, omissions, or any inconsistency herein.

Printed in the United States of America.
Library of Congress Control Number: 2019905854
ISBN: 978-1-94963-950-6, 978-1-7342583-3-2

Cover Design: Melanie Cloth
Layout Design: Jamie Wise

To Diane, Jordan, and Alexis: For your inspiration, love, and support.

TABLE OF CONTENTS

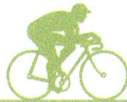

CHAPTER ONE

BETTER, FASTER, STRONGER AS YOU AGE? WHO'S WITH ME?

D oes any of this sound familiar?

You're exhausted and can't wait to get home and relax. "Exercise now? You're kidding!" you say. You don't even know what you're having for dinner.

Your sex drive is as tired as you are!

You need your reading glasses to see what someone is showing you. Worse yet, you can't remember where you left them!

You wake up during the night, not always to pee. What's up with that?

When you do wake up, it's five o'clock in the morning and your brain is whirling with worries and things to do, and you can't relax and fall back to sleep.

You can't get rid of that tire around your waist. You've read about five different diet plans in the last month, and you're not sure which to follow or believe. Nothing that you've tried in the past has worked or kept the weight off.

Your doctor has informed you that your cholesterol is high and you should start taking a statin drug. If that's not enough, you're prediabetic too.

You're trying to increase your exercise but can't get past your current walking or running time.

You're struggling to remember the name of that guy ...

Only someone middle aged and beyond can relate to these issues. Don't be embarrassed! Get excited! I'm going to use what I have learned in two and a half decades as a medical doctor to coach you through the maze of confusing information and show you a practical approach to a healthier lifestyle for all ages, but especially middle age and beyond. I've got a plan for you.

It's a healthy lifestyle program—including nutrition, exercise, and mindfulness—for anyone who wants to keep hammering it forever. And I will show you the medical science behind this program. We will also review cardiac risk factors, hormonal replacement, and sleep.

If you're a weekend warrior and wondering how we improve the performance of world-class elite endurance athletes, such as Tour de France bikers, I'll teach you—and show how to apply it to you. Say you're proud of your last 10K race time, but you know you could do better. Or you'd like to tackle a longer run, but don't have any steam left after six miles. You might wonder what tests we perform on top athletes, and how we use the results to improve their race times. You'd like to know what adjustments we make to an endurance athlete's diet, and how we determine how much they should eat before, during, and after the race.

You may be primarily interested in health and wellness, and preventive medicine or antiaging techniques. What is the healthiest, research-supported nutrition program? I've got it for you. No more struggles to lose weight or keep it off. Seriously. This is a long-term victory.

My career in medicine has focused on caring for people who are getting older. I've seen tens of thousands of men and women in my office over the decades and have closely observed what happens to them as they age.

A few years ago, I did a fellowship in antiaging medicine at a practice called Cenegenics in Las Vegas. I later opened and ran the firm's Boulder, Colorado, facility as its medical director. My passion for fitness and healthy eating has led me to study and learn from the medical literature and great experts.

As I watched my patients fall into various cycles of decline, I kept asking: is there a better way? There is. I have developed a program and a plan for you. I will share my knowledge and insights.

• • •

"Don't get old, Dr. Ehrlich!" Patients told me this regularly during my early years of medical practice in Venice, Florida. Their arthritic knees and other ailments were overwhelming them, making them believe there was nothing to do to stop the negative effects of aging.

They were wrong. I will train you to reduce the deterioration of the human body that I have seen regularly in my patients. One of my goals: to keep you out of the operating rooms of heart surgeons, orthopedists, or other doctors. If I can safeguard you from having to go through invasive medical procedures or surgery, it will be well worth the price of admission.

But let's try to set the bar higher than keeping the doctor away. First, I want to be clear about what I am not promising. It's not within my power to add years to your life. I also can't bring you back the youthful looks you had in your thirties. Nor can I offer you a flat belly overnight, as some faddish diet gurus promise.

If you sign on to the plan I outline in these pages—and stick with it—it will help you lose that weight and keep it off, without "dieting"; improve and maintain your fitness; and achieve a heightened state of energy, eagerness for life, emotional passion for loved ones, and peace of mind. These are things that often elude people as they grow older. But they are crucial to a comfortable, happy life.

And that brighter, more energetic you will likely find yourself setting new goals that you never imagined—and achieving them. For some, this will mean cutting time off your marathon. Others will find their nirvana in biking an extra hour or tackling that steep climb without feeling breathless. For some it may be a renewed energy at work, a clear mind to focus on projects and new ideas. You might be comfortable joining the ranks of my patients who even as octogenarians participate in such demanding adventures as long-distance cycling trips through Europe, or hiking and camping in yurts between Aspen and Crested Butte.

I am confident that the healthy lifestyle prescribed in my plan will bring positive results for anyone, whether they're new to healthy eating and regular exercise or more advanced in their habits.

In particular, I am committed to helping men and women who are already oriented toward a healthy lifestyle calibrate their game plan and kick it up a notch or two. With determination and some good old-fashioned work, those of you who are not there yet can join us. I'm going to show you how to do this with the latest in exercise physiology and sports nutrition.

I know that my program can inspire and guide middle-aged, seasoned fitness warriors. Michael, a Boston-based business executive in his early sixties, comes to mind. A devoted runner, he does long runs three to four times a week. And for years he has raced in the Boston Marathon. For some time now, Michael's marathon time has been stuck at around three hours fifty minutes. "Can I do better than that at my age?" he asked.

I'm going to share with you the science behind how we improve the performance of everyone from elite endurance athletes, such as bikers who compete in the Tour de France, to weekend warriors. We will also show you how we nourish them before, during, and after the competition, and how this applies to a regimen for you.

Lois, a fifty-year-old administrator in Phoenix, and Steve, a middle-aged business man, are excellent cases in point. Lois tries to exercise, but she's stressed out with her teenagers and work. Her body weight is a bit above where she would like it to be and her cholesterol is high. She asks: "Is there a way for me to get my weight and cholesterol under control?"

Steve can't quiet his mind. He awakes at night, and rather than falling back to sleep his mind races with worries over money, aggravation at work, or disagreements with his wife. He's overweight and hasn't exercised in a while. At work, his creativity has stagnated. Steve suffers from depression and anxiety and would benefit from the exercise and mindfulness that I preach.

In these cases—and so many others like them—my plan can help. It can guide Michael, Lois, and Steve to build on the clear dedication that they have to fitness and wellness and usher them toward their higher goals. And it can help you, too!

• • •

I call my plan the Vail Method. The name was inspired by Vail, the Colorado town near where my family and I make our home. An alluring village located in the Rocky Mountains, Vail is known as a top international ski destination.

For those of us who live here, Vail's biggest draw is as an enclave offering a positive and healthy lifestyle for everyone, including those of us who are fifty and older. My neighbors and I enjoy a variety of sports year-round: running, hiking, biking, and skiing. The glorious mountains and pristine air beg for exploration in every season.

Healthy eating is also part of the Vail way of life. Colorado is farm rich, providing the basis for a steady inflow of fresh local products.

I will sing the praises of Vail much more in chapter 2. But let me summarize the high points of the Vail Method here. It has four core aspects:

1. plant-based diet and nutrition

2. aerobic exercise with lactate threshold testing and heart rate-based training

3. rest, with avoidance of overtraining, and adequate sleep

4. mindfulness and relaxation

Good nutrition and maintaining a desirable body weight are key goals of the Vail Method.

Nutrition can be a confusing topic even for those of us with a keen professional interest in it. The wide range of views on the subject can make you dizzy. Anyone can propose a diet and be an expert. There is no training or education required to do so. As a result, the array of diets being promoted is vast: plant-based versus paleo, keto, low carb, gluten free, and so on. How does one choose?

Most medical doctors are not that informed about nutrition. But some of my colleagues and I are passionately involved and can use our scientific rigor and medical background to help you.

One thing I can do, for starters, is help separate myth from science in the areas of diet and exercise. As anyone who has researched best practices in diet or exercise knows, the information out there is often contradictory. One "expert" says never eat avocados because they're high in saturated fat. Another advises eating avocados as a source of healthy fat that helps you maintain your weight. Years of work as a doctor help me guide you to adopt and follow habits that are supported by science—ones that really work.

My analyses of studies, coupled with personal experiences over many years, have led me to conclude that a plant-based diet with whole grains and whole, unprocessed food is the hands-down winner for preventing heart disease, the leading killer in the US. Plant-based diets also work best for reducing the risk of cancer, losing weight, and combating high blood sugar.

Thus, following a 100 percent vegetarian diet—or one that is close enough and still fits in your comfort zone—is a cornerstone of the Vail Method.

Chapters 4 and 5 will explore the health benefits of a plant-based diet and will explain how to transition to one in a Western world of primarily meat eaters. It will include basics on nutrients in food, and the amounts of carbohydrates and protein you need, with guidelines for sports nutrition. In chapter 5, I will focus on how to make a plant-based diet practical for you. You will see examples of various grain and bean serving sizes and how many calories, carbohydrates, and protein are in these servings. This will help guide you in preparing meals and portions. And I will touch on the toxic world of food—which, regardless of what diet you follow, is the next battleground of the twenty-first century.

Chapter 4 will share the research that led me to favor a plant-based diet. The approach I use is known as evidence-based medicine. That refers to recommendations based on sound clinical trials from peer-reviewed medical journals in which teams of experts review the study and the findings for scientific validity. In other words, there is a solid body of scientific research behind the Vail Method.

One important point: while I believe that sticking with a diet is crucial, I also recognize that we have to leave some wiggle room. We humans are social creatures. We need to be able to go out to eat and have fun with friends, and sometimes plant-based options are not available or extremely limited. Travel sometimes makes it hard to stick strictly to any eating plan. Some flexibility in what you eat is key.

For instance, during a recent ten-day vacation with my family to Paris and London, finding restaurants that suited everyone's diet and palate was not always easy. While at home I stick to a plant-based diet, during the trip I found myself eating some fish, dairy products, more French bread than whole grains, and fewer veggies then normal, often prepared with butter and oils.

Aerobic exercise is another crucial component of the Vail Method. A consistent regime of running, biking, hiking, or swimming—or a combination of these—is important to attaining and maintaining an adequate fitness level.

To get the best cardiac benefit for you, we'll start by pinpointing your experience and comfort level with aerobic activities. What kind of fitness regime do you follow? Not exercising at all? Once a week? Or four times a week? And for how long?

And then we'll do some tests. I describe the various scientific examinations you will need in chapter 3. By far the most important is the exam to determine your training heart rate. This is an area in which research has made great advances in recent years. Even for veteran runners or bikers, calibrating your fitness at the start will make a big difference. It will help us design the most effective workout routine to obtain better results.

The old formulas for maximum heart rates—still used on some watches and treadmills—at best only provide rough estimates, and often poor ones, leading to incorrect ranges for your target heart rate for exercise. For Vail Method devotees, I recommend lactate threshold testing, the state-of-the-art approach for determining this. I'll explain the test in chapter 3, and how we use the results to optimize your routine in chapter 6.

You will need a heart monitor with a watch that records your heart rate and the length of your workout. The watch should have built-in GPS so you can record the distance that you walk or run, as well as the pace.

Years ago, when I started using my first monitor, I thought it would be a novelty that I would use a few times to see what my heart rate was, and then my interest would wane. To the contrary, I now use my heart rate and pace as coaching tools. It shows me when I'm not working hard enough (or too hard), so I will pick up the pace, or slow down.

Another recommendation: keep a diary to record your aerobic workouts. In our electronic world this is so easy. You can track all kinds of information about exercise: Did you run or bike or swim? Were you tired, or did you feel good? Did you drink coffee for a caffeine boost?

Now, time to get moving! You are likely an experienced runner.

But, if you're new to aerobic exercise, walking is a good place to start. You'll need to walk for a longer time than you would run to get a good effect. If you're moving more slowly than a twelve-minute mile, which is a brisk walk, then try to go for an hour a day. Any hills or inclines will add work and benefit.

For those who prefer biking or swimming, we have regimens for you too. The important thing is to choose an aerobic exercise that you're comfortable engaging in over the long haul, or mix them up with cross training.

I am aware that some trainers recommend a treadmill over trail running, particularly for those over fifty. But I have a strong bias toward outdoor walking and running. Why? While you can raise your heart rate on a treadmill, the muscular effort is not the same. On a treadmill, you simply need to keep up with a motorized moving belt. This does not compare to the energy and effort required to lift your body off the ground with each foot strike when running outside. A treadmill, elliptical machine, or stationary bike also does not challenge your core muscles to balance you on each stride or pedal stroke. If you are using a treadmill, raise the incline to at least one percent to more closely mimic running outdoors.

How many times a week should you do an aerobic workout? Kenneth Cooper, MD, one of the fathers of aerobic exercise, impressed me years ago with his medical data. He first recommended aerobic exercise three times per week for at least twenty minutes. Once you achieve a healthy fitness level, this is a good way to maintain it. The off days allow your body to recover from minor strains and pains.

For those trying to get in shape, more frequent workouts are necessary in the beginning, and in fairness, these workouts are usually less intense. So, beginners should plan to walk an hour every day if possible.

One warning: if you only exercise three times a week, you have to be diligent about your workout schedule. If one day comes that you have a reason to skip—bad weather, lack of sleep, a commitment at work or home, bad juju—suddenly you find that your workout is now four days from your last effort.

Besides aerobic exercise, you should train with weights on a regular basis. A weight training or Pilates regime is essential to maintaining muscle mass, which we can lose as we age.

It's standard knowledge that a *good night's sleep* is another huge component of a healthy life. Without a long, consistent night of solid sleep, none of the other aspects of the Vail Method will be fully effective. Yet, sound sleep is something that eludes many of us. Sometimes sleep apnea is to blame.

Over the years, at countless social outings, I have heard friends and acquaintances make comments about their sleep. Generally, the conversation follows one of a few common threads: how loudly their spouse snores; the number of times they wake up in the night, either to urinate or because of shortness of breath or other, unknown reasons; or how early they wake up.

Many of these complaints are not normal, "just getting older" aspects of aging. They are caused by sleep apnea. What is that? As we age, the soft palate in the roof of our mouths relaxes. When we lie on our backs, our tongue slides back in our mouths and occludes our airway. We literally are choking when this occurs. Our blood oxygen saturation decreases. The lack of oxygen causes us to wake up so we will change position and get some air.

My point here is to introduce the concept of sleep apnea and make you aware that you may be afflicted with it. If you are, you can't restore your body as you need to with sleep. This causes your day to begin in a negative spiral, since you can't exercise well if you're exhausted. Or you will simply find an excuse to skip exercise. This in turn completes the whole cycle of problems that keep you from achieving the fitness you desire, a suitable weight, and the good health that you want to have as you age.

Fortunately, there are effective ways to address sleep apnea. I will review the testing in chapter 3 and treatment options in chapter 9.

An active sex life, too, is a feature of the healthy lifestyle I promote. Just reading the word *sex* probably woke you up! Now let's have an open and honest conversation about the topic. From the millions spent on Viagra and Cialis commercials you know that something is going on with our sex lives as we grow older. Does every man over fifty have erectile dysfunction, often referred to as ED? Is it an epidemic? On the rise (no pun intended)? Do women over fifty lose their sex drive too?

The reality: with age, sex hormone levels drop for men and women. Sorry guys! Women go through perimenopause, then menopause. One thing discussed much less in our sexist world is that after men reach the age of forty, we go through "andropause" as our testosterone levels drop. It's becoming more acceptable to talk about "low T" for men who suffer from this. Still, traditional family medicine fails to regularly measure testosterone levels in men, and even more importantly infrequently attempts to treat it.

So, among other tests, I recommend having your testosterone measured. Reliable treatments are available and accessible for both men and women with low levels. A normal physiological testosterone level will make it easier to build or maintain muscle mass, lose weight, and have the energy and zest for life and sex you had when you were younger.

Mindfulness is another core component of our lifestyle regime and is the topic of chapter 8. To tackle our daily to-do lists with clarity and without feeling overwhelmed, we all need to find some way to focus and calm the mind. In my experience, mindfulness is a highly individualistic pursuit. In the mountainous part of Colorado where I live, many find solace in nature walks. For others, mediation is helpful. Still others find a centeredness in the church or personal spirituality.

This is an area of the Vail Method where no one approach is more effective than another, although medical research is showing some amazing health benefits from meditation. The important thing is to recognize the value of mindfulness and to find a way to engage in it that works for you.

The Vail Method is a practical, holistic approach, a "how to" guide, using scientifically proven, evidence-based medicine. Think of it as an owner's guide to the human body. By holistic, I am not referring to herbal supplements, but rather a comprehensive guide to aging well and remaining strong.

The Vail Method engages so many aspects of your life that ulti-mately signing onto it is a lifestyle choice. Maintaining a consistent, healthy diet will call on you to devote time to shopping right and thought to preparing nutritious meals that include plant protein. Keeping up a regular exercise regime will require you to allocate three to four hours a week and, in some cases, more.

But the first action required of you is an internal one. You must ask yourself if you're committed to changing your habits. This may be the hardest question to answer honestly. How honestly, you ask? Think of the way that your teenage children or grandchildren challenge you to talk about how you really are—the kind of candid, loving truth that gets to the heart of the matter.

Sticking to this new lifestyle will involve commitment. You have to be truly devoted to it. And because there are only so many hours in the day, that inevitably means choosing priorities and making sacrifices. There will be times when you may have to pull yourself away from a gathering of friends or other activities to get a run in. Over time, making a healthy lifestyle a high priority will become easier and more natural.

Signing onto the Vail Method may also change the dynamic of your relationship with your spouse or life partner. To make this work, it helps to have an accepting co-conspirator. Success over the long haul will be easier if you have someone close who embraces the priorities you give to this approach to eating and exercising. Better yet would be one who buys into the program and its benefits as much as you do. That would give you a constant workout partner and a dining companion who shares your commitment. Also, some of us have the self-discipline to exercise alone, maintain the frequency, and enjoy the solace. But for others it is easier to involve friends socially in physical activities, from biking or jogging together to gym classes.

In many cases, engaging a partner in this new lifestyle will be tough. My wife of more than thirty years does not share my approach to diet or exercise. But she has given me support and the freedom and time to indulge it and has creatively worked to develop recipes for the vegetarians and meat eaters alike in our family.

• • •

I am confident that the goals in the Vail Method are achievable because I have attained them.

I "walk the talk"—and run and cycle. I follow a plant-based diet, with some exceptions, as I mentioned above. Even in my late fifties, I regularly compete in races. Earlier this year, in fitness-oriented Boulder, Colorado, I took fifth place for my age in a field of fifty thousand runners in the popular Bolder Boulder 10K. A few months later, after a summer of longer runs, I tackled the Rock 'n' Roll Denver Half Marathon, a distance I have not raced in ages. I was pleased to finish in tenth place for my age group.

So, let me help you and let's work together.

As you learn more about the medical consequences of an unhealthy diet and lifestyle, you will realize how one problem connects to the next—like a rolling snowball speeding down the hill—or can be stopped in its tracks by good habits as prescribed in the Vail Method.

If you follow an unhealthy diet and fail to exercise, you are likely to be overweight. The repercussions of this go beyond appearance and energy. You are more likely to have the metabolic syndrome or diabetes. Your risk for stroke or heart attack and death are higher.

But there is good news: it's never too late to start fresh or ramp up your game.

Let's get on the right track now.

CHAPTER TWO

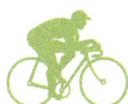

RUN, BIKE, HIKE, SKI: THE MECCA OF VAIL

t was a Saturday morning in summer and I had just ascended Bellyache Ridge, a steep paved road with grades from 5 to 13 percent in the Vail Valley of Colorado. I had climbed more than two thousand vertical feet on my trusted road bike. It took an hour and it was so worth it. The view from an overlook near the top was nothing short of stunning. The mountain peaks glistened in the sun, and the Eagle River twisted its way across the valley floor.

On the way down, I circled into the Red Sky Golf Course, about a mile from the bottom of the climb. From there, I began ascending another winding road for seven hundred vertical feet. I stopped to admire an awesome view of the golf course and the golfers teeing up and swinging away.

That's when it hit me. It was magical mornings like this—doing hard-driving exercise in a picture-perfect natural setting—that inspired the Vail Method. In fact, the roots of a fitness program especially tailored for middle agers on up had been growing in my mind and soul for some time.

For years I have followed an intensely health-oriented lifestyle. That has meant sticking religiously to healthy eating habits that have evolved into a plant-based diet. It has also involved regular, focused aerobic exercise—running and cycling. And it has included a commitment to mindfulness, the focused practice of calming the mind and spirit. The natural splendor of my environment, the Vail Valley, connects all these elements seamlessly.

This lifestyle has worked well for my own health, well-being, and spirit, and I wanted to share it with others, especially those already dedicated to exercise and healthy eating. Using my own fitness and diet regime as the basis, I devised a program that could help guide others in their later forties and up to achieve an elevated level of physical and mental rejuvenation. It took being out on my bike in the Vail Valley to realize that the time was now to bring the parts of the Vail Method together and introduce them to folks like you.

This region—with its mix of big sky, fresh air, and easy access to outdoor pursuits—is a logical place to launch such a lifestyle change. Spending some time in Vail and the surrounding area can help as you get started on the Method—or even after you are well into it. Vail offers an impressive range of recreational opportunities. Those of you who are versatile in sports can experience what we call a Vail trifecta. That refers to participating in different sports or recreational activities in the course of a single day. Depending on the activities you enjoy, in the early spring, it could be skiing in the morning, a bike ride at noon, and fishing or nine holes of golf in the afternoon. Yes, welcome to Vail and the fitness and recreational enthusiasts who live here.

Another big draw to our area is the camaraderie. As an active middle-aged athlete—or aspiring athlete—who is committed to running, biking, and other types of exercise, you will be in good company in Vail and the surrounding area. Our year-round residents include a core percentage of men and women in their fifties and older. Group runs and bike rides are publicized in the local paper, coffee shops, and bike and running stores. Added to that are quite a few people who summer or winter here on a regular basis—and many of them are big recreation fans. In summer, it's not unusual to see a group of middle-aged and older men and women cycling along the mountain roads. And of course, come winter, skiers of all ages congregate here.

But you don't need to come to Colorado—or travel anywhere—to embrace the Vail Method and make it part of your life. In fact, I am sure most of you will launch the program from your home base. I have designed every step so that you can start and stay engaged, whether you are New York City or Des Moines.

As I outline the various aspects of the Vail Method throughout the book, I will describe ways to make the plan accessible wherever you are. In chapter 3 I discuss a variety of exams—from a general physical to a lactate threshold test—recommended for anyone starting the program. Your family doctor can handle some of these tests. A lactate test at a center with experience is more difficult to find. Exercise laboratories associated with some universities are a place to start looking. In chapter 5, I talk about how to create a plant-based diet regime. You can find all the ingredients you need at your local supermarket or online. The exercise regimes that I detail in chapter 6 are all possible to do on running or bike trails or gyms near your home.

Even though the different aspects of the Vail Method—regular aerobic exercise, a plant-based diet, mindfulness, rest, and so on—

are individual pursuits, it helps to engage in them with other like-minded people. This is particularly true for those of you who do not have partners or family who are joining you in the Vail Method.

For running, Vail offers many varieties of terrain and settings. You might stride along a recreation path that follows the Eagle River, or a three- to four-foot-wide creekside dirt path that runs along the valley floor with views of the mountains on both sides. Near my house is a paved road that has a nice eighteen-inch dirt shoulder; it goes by horse farms with deer that run from one side to the other, hop a fence, and sprint off, bounding across the field. Or you might spot a red fox or herd of elk.

Trail running is popular in Vail. These trails are sometimes shared with mountain bikers on the ski mountains or in the community trail area. But sometimes there are runners only. Uphill trail running is a great cardio workout that also will build your strength.

Biking options abound in spring, summer, and early fall until the snow starts falling and the temperatures plummet. Both road cycling and mountain biking are beloved among locals and visitors. Our road conditions are quite good, something I have learned to appreciate when riding on roads elsewhere in the US.

If some of the bike rides I describe above sound intense, consider the group of fanatics who bike the Octopus, a local ride held once each year. In this race, the Bellyache Ridge ride is only one of eight similar climbs. Since we have no ocean to see a real octopus, we apply that name to a route that has eight legs similar to the ride I described above, but only done in a series, all in one day! A support van from one of the local bike shops follows the riders, offering water refills and snacks to keep them going.

If you are not yet a road cyclist, I'd like to see you work on acquiring the essential skills of road biking, especially descending hills at higher speeds. As with any new skill it will take some time and effort, but it's good to challenge your mind and body by learning new tasks. And once you experience the hard cardio work of climbing uphill and the thrill of winding down the hill, taking small curves or "switchbacks" to slow your speed to a comfortable pace, feeling the acceleration of the curve as it takes you gently around a bend, you will be hooked.

Besides the thrills, there are obvious fitness benefits. At these elevated altitudes we generate more red blood cells because the oxygen in our air is thinner, and we need more cells to circulate and carry oxygen. This aids in training for when we go down to sea level and feel like we have an oxygen tank to supply us.

Our idea of a great road bike ride in Vail is to go up paved roads on mountains as we track our gain in vertical feet from the base where we started to the top of the ride. Often a ride like this will have a gain of at least two thousand vertical feet over four to five miles. These relentless climbing rides will have pitches averaging close to 8 percent with some stretches exceeding 10 percent.

Downhill skiing is a popular pursuit at the renowned Vail Mountain. But you might not have considered the various types of skiing that are much more fitness-oriented and relevant to the Vail Method.

Cross-country skiing takes place on groomed trails with a "classic" course. More exciting is skate skiing, in which the skier uses ice skating-like movements to move quickly along the path, as seen in the winter Olympic races. Once again, our hilly terrain adds to the workout, and most cross-country ski areas offer flat courses as well as some that go up and down relatively small hills, enough to get your heart going. Many people enjoy the solitude and experience of cross-country skiing in remote areas.

Less known to most who don't reside in ski country is "AT," or "all terrain" skiing. In Vail we call it "skinning," which refers to the material bands made of mohair or other fibers that we stick to the bottom of the AT ski to give it traction as we glide up the mountain. The AT ski bindings are special as well, with adjustments that allow them to lift up and glide when going uphill, then lock down for more support like a regular ski binding to ski down. We carry backpacks with extra layers to wear for warmth if needed on the descent, and dress more lightly than you might expect for the outdoor temperature to minimize getting wet and sweaty on the ascent. AT skiing is allowed at certain times at the ski resorts and at parks and paths in Vail, including backcountry areas. But because of avalanche danger in the backcountry, it's best to go only with one of our experienced guides.

For hikers, the nearby mountains have hut systems that enable overnight hiking. In winter or summer, hikers sleep in yurts and move on to the next yurt the following day.

Other active pursuits include ice climbing in winter, rock climbing in summer, and whitewater rafting in spring. As our temperatures heat up and snow stops falling, the snowmelt from the mountains runs down into the rivers, creating Class IV rapids in sections of the Eagle River. In June, the water temperature is about fifty degrees, so one does not want to be a "swimmer" who falls out of the raft. But with our professional guides this is rare, and safety measures are in place to keep it from happening.

Another thing that enhances the aura of Vail as a recreation destination is that it is home to world-class athletes who engage in most of the activities described above. We also are fortunate to have world-renowned orthopedic surgeons pursuing both clinical and basic science research, including stem cell work.

In addition, our physical therapists supporting the community of athletes are superb. They help keep many of us out of surgery by assessing muscular weaknesses that contribute to imbalances and injuries, then developing programs for us to strengthen these weaknesses. For runners, many of our problems relate to weak gluteal muscles. Good physical therapists will show you how to strengthen these muscles. That, too, is part of the Vail Method and will be covered in detail in chapter 6.

CHAPTER THREE

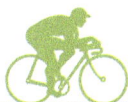

THE TESTS YOU NEED NOW

Years of treating patients have shown me that every person has unique physical capabilities, strengths, and limits. Some folks in their fifties and up, with rigorous training, can finish marathons in under three hours. Others can do hard, driving gym workouts, deftly moving from bench presses to squats and pull-ups, with intense aerobic intervals mixed in. Still others are ultra-endurance 100-mile runners.

I have learned that whatever our limits seem to be, we can stretch them further. For most of us, building to a level of peak athletic performance requires time and training. The Vail Method is designed to help you evaluate your physical strengths and weaknesses. I will then guide you to expanding your capabilities—in the gym, on the running trail, or on your road or mountain bike—to achieve higher levels of performance.

First, some tests are in order. Poking and prodding can be a bit of a pain, I know. But the information we obtain from these tests will be instrumental in putting you on the right path to improved health and fitness.

Before we get to these tests, we need to make sure that your physical health is strong. If you have not undergone a complete yearly exam with your primary care physician, I encourage you to do so. Make sure it includes the essential tests and measures: routine blood work, urinalysis, blood pressure, weight, and oxygen saturation of the blood.

Four additional exams in particular are essential to the Vail Method. A lactate threshold test is probably the most important. It will guide us in creating the best aerobic workout regime for you. A testosterone test for men and women will inform us if you suffer from low testosterone, which drains your energy levels, sex drive, and ability to shed body fat and maintain muscle mass. For women, additional hormonal tests are needed as discussed below. A body fat test will allow us to determine your fat versus lean body mass. With this information, we can track your progress and determine if you need to adjust your diet. A fourth very useful test is an ultrasound of your muscles that will show us your glycogen stores and give us insight into your nutritional status, including how well you replace your calories and carbohydrates after exercise.

Depending on the particular health issues you are dealing with, some other exams might be in order. Struggling with sleep? It would be a good idea to take a sleep apnea test. Having hip or back issues? Our physical therapists can assess your weaknesses and help design a program to relieve your pain and get you back to your best form for sports. Also, in some cases, a running gait analysis or bike fit evaluation could help. Worried about your risk of heart attack? There are a couple of useful assessments you can do. For some of you, this category of tests is optional. I will offer some pointers that will help you determine whether they are necessary and how they might help.

If the range and focus of these exams seem broad, it is because the spirit behind the Vail Method is holistic and all-encompassing. I am interested in nurturing and improving everything about your health, from your posture while you are running to how your brain works.

Make sure that you record the results of all the tests and keep them organized, preferably in an online diary or a binder in your file cabinet. Later chapters will discuss how to put the information we obtain from the test results to good use. In chapter 6, which is devoted to honing your workouts, I walk you through how to use the results of the lactate threshold test and running gait or biking analyses.

LACTATE THRESHOLD TESTING

To help you understand why the lactate threshold test is so crucial, let me offer a mini-lesson in cell biology. Lactic acid is formed when muscle cells convert glucose into energy. *Lactate threshold* is basically the intensity of exercise at which lactic acid begins to accumulate in the blood at a faster rate than it can be removed. In all of our cells there is an organelle known as the mitochondria that takes the lactate and revitalizes it to get rid of the lactic acid. It turns out that those mitochondria are pretty important in determining athletic performance. Researchers have conducted muscle biopsies on athletes and sedentary patients and found out some fascinating things. High-performing athletes such as Tour de France cyclists have big, fat, juicy mitochondria, and many more of them than recreational athletes.

In sedentary, overweight people, the mitochondria look sad and shrunken, and their numbers are far fewer than in their exercising, age-matched peers.

Figure 3.1 is a photo showing muscle biopsies of obese patients before and after a university-supervised, sixteen-week program of exercise and weight loss through caloric restriction.[1] They completed two exercise sessions per week at 60-70 percent of maximum heart rate. The muscle fibers are seen as uniform and striped in appearance. Between the muscle fibers is the intermyofibrillar spaces, where you can see small dark spots, or glycogen, and larger black circles, which are the mitochondria. Note the enlargement of the mitochondria following the exercise program. This correlated with an increase in exercise performance, known as VO2 max, from 39 to 46.

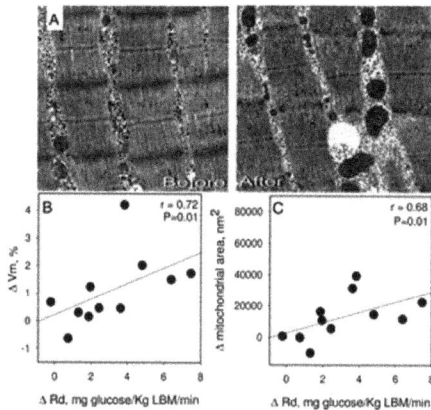

Figure 3.1: Obese patients' muscle biopsies.

From: Changes Induced by Physical Activity and Weight Loss in the Morphology of Intermyofibrillar Mitochondria in Obese Men and Women. J Clin Endocrimnal Metab. 2008; 91(8): 3224-3227. doi: 10.1210/ jc.2008-0002. J Clin Endocrinal Metab | Copyright © 2006 by The Endocrine Society

Mitochondrial health, or the lack of it, also has important consequences for glucose metabolism, plays a role in diabetes and even abnormal brain glucose metabolism, and has a possible connection to Alzheimer's disease. As you can see, it is critical to build up your mitochondria. Knowing your lactate threshold will help us, or whoever is doing the lactate test, to create a customized program designed to increase mitochondrial size and density.

To begin you wear a heart monitor strap and a mask to measure your exhaled gases, as you are positioned on a treadmill. Before you start, the examiner will get a baseline lactate level via a finger stick that draws a small drop of blood from your fingertip. This lactate level normally is around 1.0 if you are at rest.

Every five minutes we will increase the speed of the treadmill and prick your finger to measure your lactate level. When your muscles begin to tire, you will feel the lactate level rise in your body. On a run, this is when you realize that you don't have much left in you. When you run out of steam on the treadmill, this is when your lactate level has risen significantly.

I have a story about my first test. Inigo San Millan, PhD, the exercise physiologist, was in the room. His assistant was getting my blood samples and adjusting the treadmill speeds. As I was wearing a mask to catch the expired gases in my breath, I couldn't talk. The assistant gave me a hand signal to alert him about how tired I was getting. One finger meant "not tired at all," while ten fingers meant "I'm exhausted."

Once the test was going, I was pushing myself. My lactate levels were being measured, but I didn't know what they were. At one point, the assistant asked me how I was doing. I put up three fingers. I knew I was understating my condition, but I wanted to continue and do as well as I could. He looked at me, and said knowingly, "Don't lie to me! I've got your blood tests right here." I suppose you had to be there to appreciate the humor, but even breathing hard with the mask on, I couldn't help but chuckle. So, I held up five fingers. I was getting close to the end, and he knew it. Even though I was still running strong on the treadmill, my blood lactate level told him the truth.

We have learned that we need to measure lactate thresholds based on your preferred activity. If you are primarily a cyclist, we would do the test on a resistance bike. If you are a runner, on a treadmill. If you do both regularly, you would need to test separately for each exercise on separate days. A specially adapted swimming pool is used to test swimmers.

A graph of lactate threshold testing and heart rate zones is shown in Figure 3.2. We see that as heart rate (the blue line) increases, lactate levels (the red line) begin to rise. The increasing workload during exercise is shown on the X axis as the speed of the treadmill in miles per hour.

When the rate of lactate removal cannot keep up with the rate of lactate production, lactate accumulates. This is shown on the Y axis on the right side of the figure. The Y axis on the left is the heart rate. We will return to this graph in more detail in chapter 6 to learn more about how we use this information to determine your target heart rate for exercise.

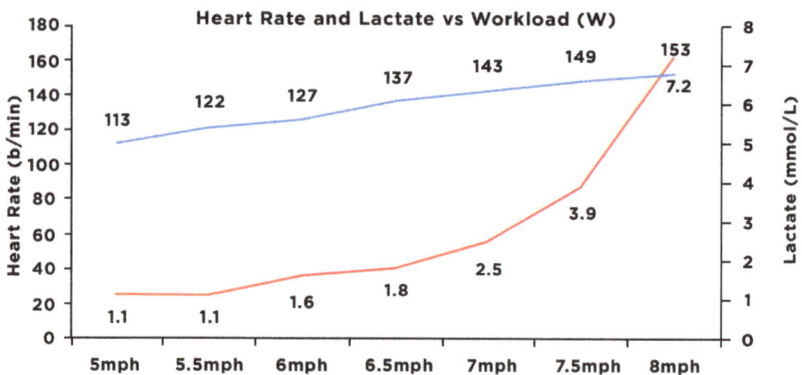

Figure 3.2: Heart rate and blood lactate level.

BODY FAT ANALYSIS

Finding out how much body fat you have is also essential. It is needed to determine your percent body fat—how much of your weight is fat and how much is lean muscle, bone, and internal organs. Of course, it will also tell us if you are overweight and, if so, by how much. We will use this data to calculate your nutritional requirements such as daily calories, protein, and carbohydrates. I walk you through that process in chapter 4. Knowing your body fat and lean muscle mass also will give us important data to monitor. For example, if we are seeing people losing weight, is it just fat they are reducing? Or are they losing lean muscle mass as well? The latter is undesirable.

There are five different ways to measure body fat. The most precise method uses Archimedes' principle—basically how much water your body displaces when submerged in a tank of water. Unfortunately, this approach is not easily available to most people. The second technique is a DXA (dual energy X-ray absorptiometry) scan. It measures the calcium in your bones to screen for osteoporosis as well as your body fat percentage. The third method involves a newer device, the Bod Pod, where a patient sits in an enclosed eggshell-shaped chamber. The volume of air displaced by the patient is used to calculate body density, which in turn is used in formulas for gender, age, and race to estimate the percentage of body fat.

Fourth, there are electronic gadgets that try to measure the conduction of a weak electric current that passes more quickly through body water and muscle than through bones and fat. This is the method used by home scales that record your weight and percentage of body fat, and other similar gadgets. It is the least reliable method. Finally, you can have a qualified technician do it, using calipers to pinch the excess skin and subcutaneous fat at your waist, hips, belly button, and so on. This is a reliable and inexpensive procedure. It's the one we use most often in the Vail Method. We encourage you to take stock of and record your percent body fat at regular intervals to make sure that you're losing fat and not muscle.

I'm often asked what percentage body fat is healthy. A range of normal or ideal is more helpful than a single number. As a general rule, healthy women should have a higher percentage of body fat than men. Most men should aim for a range from 15 to 18 percent up to 20 percent. That said, elite cyclists normally range from 10 to 15 percent. Women should aim for a range of 15 to 25 percent. There have been some reports of elite female athletes who achieved 10 percent. But we caution against such low levels. In this range, we can see problems with menstrual function and other health concerns.

ULTRASOUND TEST FOR MUSCLE GLYCOGEN

Dr. San Millan developed an innovative muscle ultrasound test that measures muscle glycogen storage. Done in lieu of a traditional muscle biopsy, this ultrasound has been shown to correlate closely with biopsy results.[2] Many factors can decrease muscle storage of glycogen, including recent exercise, overseas travel, and most importantly inadequate carbohydrate and calorie consumption by the athlete. Inadequate carbohydrate consumption has been a problem over the years because of nonexperts advising people that "carbs are bad for you."

Taking this test is easy. You will lie down on a table and an ultrasound probe will be rubbed from your pelvis to your kneecap along your quadriceps, focusing on the rectus femoris muscle. A lubricating jelly is on the bottom of the ultrasound probe. There is no discomfort to the test. Ultrasound imaging is the technology used to see a baby in a pregnant woman's womb.

HORMONES

Hormones are another topic to consider. After we reach the age of forty, men's and women's sex hormones begin falling significantly. Low testosterone affects male and female mood and energy, libido, ability to maintain muscle mass—which is an issue as we age—and ability to lose excess body fat.

For women, the hormonal landscape is much more complicated than for men. For you to feel and be your best, we need to understand the symptoms you are having as the result of changing levels of your thyroid hormone, estrogen, progesterone, and cortisol. They all interact in a complicated hormonal soup.

The testosterone and other hormonal tests are something that your doctor should do. They can be added to your blood work during a regular checkup. A thyroid test would normally be done with routine lab tests. Women should also request that a physician check their estrogen and progesterone levels. When testing for testosterone levels, it is important to measure the free or available testosterone. It gets attached to a binding protein, such that total testosterone levels can be normal, but with high binding proteins "free T" may actually be low.

The typical treatment for low testosterone in men is an injection, administered once a week, in the muscle of your rear end. What is an optimal testosterone level for a man? There is a wide range of normal, from three hundred to more than one thousand. Cenegenics, the company where I worked, specializes in testosterone supplementation. A reasonable limit for total testosterone is around five hundred to six hundred, which gives you the boost you need but not up to superman levels.

If women are experiencing deficiencies, a gynecologist will usually prescribe bio identical hormones, including creams for testosterone and pills or creams for estrogen and progesterone. With women, levels are different, and they need to avoid excess testosterone treatment. In our program, we rely on doctors who specialize in treating women and have special interest in bio identical hormones.

Some people think that treatment of low testosterone in men directly addresses erectile dysfunction, or ED. It does not. ED is primarily an atherosclerotic, circulatory issue, or hardening of the arteries. As the artery involved is small in diameter, ED is often considered a "canary in a coal mine" in that it demonstrates that arterial disease is already present. In fact, men with ED are at increased risk for developing heart disease. The whole topic of impotence is a complicated one involving psychological factors. Sex drive, however, will improve with testosterone replacement therapy.

RUNNING GAIT ANALYSIS AND BIKE FIT

For people suffering nagging injuries and pain that limit their ability to run and cycle, there are some additional optional tests alluded to above. The running gait analysis is one of them. The test can also be helpful for experienced runners who want to maximize their running efficiency and speed. The results can help guide you in how to use the elastic recoil of your tendons and avoid overworking your muscles. With the gait analysis we can hone on your strengths and weaknesses, then use that information to design a program of exercises to help you be a stronger, better runner.

For this test, we'll start by evaluating your muscle strength on the ground and on the exam table. It's enlightening for you to see how on one side you can do a single-leg squat, while on the other side you're swaying or struggling to hold the position and not fall over. Then we'll get you warmed up on a treadmill and record a video of you running. We'll focus on different angles, from your hips to your feet. We're looking for many things.

We're watching your whole stride, beginning with your initial contact with the ground, the midstance, and finally your push off to the next landing. How do your arms swing? Is the swing the same on both sides? How about your hips? Are they level, or is one side dropping? Runners are often curious and concerned if they are a heel striker or a midfoot striker. Much more important than what part of your foot makes contact on landing is where your foot lands in relation to your center of mass. We want it under you, not out in front. These are just a few of the things we observe in the running gait analysis. We'll discuss some solutions to common problems later in chapter 6.

While a full running gait analysis may not be necessary, having a trainer do a partial assessment of your leg and hip muscle strength and balance is usually productive. Most runners have weak gluteal muscles. The gluteus medius, for example, is important for keeping the hips balanced when running. One side will usually be weaker than another, but it can be excessively weak and need work.

Some cyclists complain of back pain during or after biking. To address this and other issues, it helps to evaluate their cycling form. There are two areas to analyze. One is the fit of your bike. We are fortunate in Vail, Boulder, and other areas in Colorado to have professional bike fitters. You should try to find one in your area. They can measure your body and determine which bike frame is best for you. Or they can take your bike and adjust the extension of the handlebar, the seat height, anterior-posterior position, and more.

Another thing to evaluate is if you are straining too much for the current strength of your gluteals to do the work and using your hip flexors instead. This can lead to lower back pain as will be explained in chapter 6. I offer exercises to strengthen your gluteal muscles in that chapter as well.

SLEEP, YOU MUST

The Vail Method also addresses the critical issue of sleep. This topic is covered in detail in chapter 9, along with the related topics of rest and avoidance of overtraining. In terms of our current discussion on testing, a sleep apnea test may be in order.

The test involves connecting wire leads taped to your chest and scalp to several monitors. It also includes an electrocardiogram (EKG) to monitor your heart rate, an oxygen saturation monitor clipped over one of your fingertips, some electroencephalogram monitors to monitor the stage and depth of your sleep and dreaming, and a nasal cannula to monitor your breathing and snoring. Leads are also connected to your legs to monitor for restless leg syndrome, or movement of your legs during sleep. A technician tracks these monitors by checking on you regularly in person and via a camera in your room.

A facility-based, hospital, or outpatient sleep laboratory-monitored study as described above is the best approach, although it is costlier. Fortunately, it is usually covered by your health insurance if your physician documents any complaints or symptoms that justify the test. One good alternative is for your physician to order home monitors, which measure several of the same parameters in the comfort of your own bed. The recording device and electrodes are shipped back to the sleep study center and the results are then analyzed and reported to your doctor. This option is much more affordable.

Although a sleep apnea test is optional, in my experience the affliction is pretty widespread. The symptoms can be debilitating, and for some people a cause of death. Sleep apnea does not allow your body to recover the way it should as you sleep. And without that recovery, the health that you want to have as you age will elude you. Fortunately, some excellent treatment options are available, including simple weight loss, a change in sleeping position, an oral appliance, and use of a continuous positive airway pressure (CPAP) machine. I discuss these options in chapter 9.

CARDIAC RISK ASSESSMENT

Although assessing your heart health is not a major focus of the Vail Method, I know that reducing the risk of heart attack is a goal for many of us as we age. Heart disease is a major killer and something many of my patients worry about. Traditional medicine promotes statin drugs as a way to lower cholesterol, which contributes to heart disease. Many of my cardiologist colleagues are taking statins, trying to reduce their LDL "bad" cholesterol as close to seventy as possible. Normally, any level less than one hundred is considered quite good. In addition to lowering bad cholesterol, statins have a good anti-inflammatory effect on blood vessels reflected in certain blood tests, such as the high-sensitivity C-reactive protein. But there are toxic effects to statins. Muscle damage, proven by biopsy, occurs from statin use, even in patients who have no muscle soreness complaints.[3] Even worse, biopsy proven studies have shown that this damage persists in patients who discontinued the drug more than a year earlier.[4] In extreme cases of muscle damage known as rhabdomyolysis, kidney damage can also occur. In addition, research has also found statins have some undesired effects on metabolism, such as raising the risk of diabetes. What's more, some patients experience reduced cognitive function or short-term memory loss, though this is more controversial. So, determining when to use statins and when not to can be a challenge.

If you are interested in risk assessment for heart attack and stroke, you should ask your doctor to add a high-sensitivity C-reactive protein and an apolipoprotein B test to the routine blood work and cholesterol panel. There is also genetic testing available for the 9P21 or "heart attack gene" as well as apolipoprotein E genotypes and KIF6 genotypes. But these are not within the scope of this book.

THE TIE BREAKER: HOW ARE YOUR ARTERIES DOING?

In clinical medicine, we often decide whether to treat patients with statin drugs based on their cholesterol levels. How do we make this decision in borderline situations? Many doctors rely on large clinical trials, where we apply the outcomes of patients with your cholesterol levels to decide if it makes sense to treat you. What is your risk of dying from a heart attack if your age is X years, your blood pressure is Y, your bad cholesterol is Z, someone in your family had a heart attack at a young age, you have a history of diabetes, etc.? Sometimes it's an easy decision, and the answer is obvious. But other times it's not. If it's a borderline situation, what's the tie breaker?

One way to approach this is to look at how your arteries are actually doing under the influence of your cholesterol, genetics, diet, and so on. Are you showing significant clogging of your arteries or not? The classic gold standard is a coronary angiogram, an invasive test that has procedural risk. This is done in more severe circumstances—when you are experiencing chest pain, for example. But most patients are unaware of some simple, noninvasive, and risk-free tests that give us a good indication of the actual state of your arteries. These are helpful in the type of routine, preventive health assessment that is relevant to our healthy lifestyle program.

One is the carotid intima-media thickness test. This is a simple ultrasound test in which a probe is held to your neck, where the carotid artery pulses. It can show cholesterol plaque in the wall of the artery, including newer, noncalcified plaque. It also measures the thickness of your inner arterial wall lining. This increases with age, so you can get a feel for how young or old your arteries are, compared to your chronological age. Our local imaging center does this test for $150.

The other is the coronary artery calcium score. This test is a CAT (CT) scan that looks for calcifications in the coronary arteries. Our hospital offers this test for $300. If you have borderline elevated cholesterol and are trying to decide whether to start a statin drug, these last two tests can provide reassurance to hold the course, particularly if you are following a plant-based diet.

CHAPTER FOUR

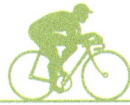

YOUR NUTRITIONAL PLAN, INCLUDING GUIDANCE FOR ENDURANCE SPORTS

A plant-based diet is a cornerstone of the Vail Method. Committing to it is an important part of maintaining great health over the long term. I've come to that conclusion after careful analysis of scientific studies by specialists whom I respect. My goal in this chapter is to share the current thinking about how a plant-based diet can help you and how it fits directly into my program.

By plant based I am speaking of a diet that consists of whole foods: primarily vegetables and fruits; whole grains like oatmeal, brown rice, and quinoa: and beans and legumes. Foods to be avoided have added sugar, refined carbohydrates, and high fat content. This will all be reviewed in detail.

Other doctors have already documented the diet-health connection; I don't want to repeat their excellent contributions but to build on them. I've also been dedicated to my own plant-based diet for years. My success with it has been remarkable and yours will be too.

I know how challenging it can be for many of you to wrap your head around a plant-based diet, let alone embrace one. Abandoning long-standing eating patterns to become vegetarian or vegan is a challenge, but an important one. The thought of sticking to kale, beans, and quinoa for the rest of your life may not sound thrilling. I get that. In reality, most of you probably believe you are already pretty healthy eaters, based on what you have learned about the standard American diet. And you're likely wondering: What's the harm of an occasional steak? Will you really get all the nutrients, especially protein, that you need from whole plant foods? These are good questions.

But the real proof in this is how much better you will feel as you enjoy more energy, weight loss, and improved blood pressure, blood sugar, and cholesterol levels.

Obviously, what you eat is up to you. But I will provide the information you need to make smart choices. For those who are skeptical about shifting to a plant-based diet, I will present some options. Finally, I'll outline an approach for changing your eating habits gradually and moderately.

The health benefits of a plant-based diet are indisputable. I've already referred to three of them: lowered rates of atherosclerotic heart disease,[5] reduced risk of cancer,[6] and longer life spans.[7] But the advantages extend far beyond this. Vegetarians are less likely to develop diabetes[8] and high blood pressure.[9] The incidence of degenerative disorders such as Parkinson's disease is also lower.[10] Vegetables contain more water and fiber than animal meats, and far more veggies can be eaten with fewer calories than the dense, high-calorie foods that comprise our typical diet. Thus, people who follow a plant-based diet weigh less, carry less fat in their tissues, and have lower rates of kidney disease. Beyond all that, plant proteins have different effects on our bodies than animal proteins and are less inflammatory to the body.[11]

Several of my colleagues in medicine have done groundbreaking work in this area and have documented their research in books. But leave it to a layman, Nathan Pritikin, to lead the way with his book *Live Longer Now*, published in 1974. He opened his Longevity Center in California one year later. And in 1977, his success with heart disease patients was chronicled by CBS's *Sixty Minutes*.

In 1978, as a medical student, Dean Ornish, MD, began work on reversing heart disease with a plant-based diet. He published his work in the medical literature[12] and in 1990, released his oft-cited book, *Dr. Dean Ornish's Program for Reversing Heart Disease: The Only System Scientifically Proven to Reverse Heart Disease without Drugs or Surgery*. A vegan, low-fat diet is at the core of his program. In 2007 Caldwell Esselstyn, MD, published a book describing his work, *Prevent and Reverse Heart Disease: The Revolutionary, Scientifically Proven, Nutrition-Based Cure*. Esselstyn, together with T. Colin Campbell, PhD, and several other contributors, produced the game-changing film, *Forks Over Knives*. It's a documentary that chronicles the plant-based diet movement. It has influenced the lives of so many, including my own.

Other colleagues have worked arduously to help disseminate this critical story. Michael Greger, MD's *How Not to Die* is a worthy read. Greger makes a strong argument for how a plant-based diet greatly diminishes our vulnerability to heart disease, cancer, and more than a dozen other chronic diseases and afflictions. In addition, his nonprofit nutritionfacts.org is a treasure trove of information. One other worthwhile volume in this genre is Garth Davis's, MD, *Proteinaholic*. Davis's book is helpful to many who are transitioning to a plant-based diet and struggling with the fear that they are not getting enough protein, as I did. He does a great job explaining our unhealthy obsession with protein. There are, of course, many others championing the cause, such as Neal Barnard, MD, John McDougall, MD, and Joel Fuhrman, MD.

As I list the many positive health effects that researchers attribute to a plant-based diet I must add this benefit: many of you will never have to engage in a weight-loss diet again. You can't put on weight from eating veggies alone. If you don't eat too much junk food such as cake, cookies, candy, or ice cream, you'll have to work hard to get enough calories from healthy foods to maintain your weight. We need to monitor you to make sure that you do so.

While adopting a plant-based diet might cause you to drop several pounds, you can be sure that you won't waste away. Your muscles won't atrophy. I worried about this myself. Could I run as fast? Bench press the same weight? You won't lose physical capacities from a plant-based diet. Quite the contrary. I promise.

How many varieties of plant-based diets are there? The terminology is confusing. Ovo-vegetarians are devoted to a plant-based diet but also eat eggs. Pesco-vegetarians include fish in their diet. Veganism is clearer, and more extreme: vegans consume no animal products, including meat, dairy products, eggs, and honey. Their mantra is simple: eat nothing that came from any creature that has a head. Veganism is what underlies most current references to a "whole-foods plant-based diet." The most extreme option in the plant-based world is an almost no-fat vegan diet, which avoids cooking oils. Even avocados are treated as bad fats. Nuts are generally frowned upon as well, except possibly a small scoop of walnuts on your oatmeal in the morning. This extreme version sometimes comes into play when confronting active heart disease where reversal, rather than just prevention, is the goal.

Deciding which of these diets best suits you is really a matter of personal taste and comfort. I question whether going to the extreme of a no-fat vegan regime is necessary for those of us not suffering from coronary artery disease. Those who opt for different variations on a plant-based diet should not be criticized by vegan enthusiasts, but welcomed to the fold. The ultimate goal is to find a place in your own journey toward a vegan plant-based diet as the ideal destination, in a way that is not a chore but feels positive and fulfilling. This kind of flexibility fits the ethos of the Vail Method.

As a general rule, I think you should eventually stick as close as possible to a plant-based diet when you are at home. There you have control over what you eat and how it is prepared. However, when you are dining out or travelling and have less control over what's put on a plate in front of you, some improvisation is in order. You have to approach such situations with a guilt-free attitude, and do what you can.

A recent example was a group biking trip in Tuscany with Backroads. We didn't just hit big tourist areas such as Siena or Florence. Instead, we were out in the country visiting smaller towns such as Rada, Montalcino, Montepulciano, and Pienza, among others. We ate at trattorias and restaurants populated with locals where the language translation assistance of our tour guides in ordering and making special requests was a big help. This gave us a real feel for the local life. It also taught me much about the Italian diet. Vegetables were plentiful, but almost always prepared with locally produced olive oil. They were delicious. Oatmeal was not available. It's not an

Italian food or custom. Of course, there is amazing homemade pasta and Italian bread. Fish is very difficult to find in the wine country of Tuscany, particularly in smaller towns. They are not close to the ocean and it is not a significant part of their diet. Steak Florentine from the local cows is popular. I did not try this. I was able to get beans, which helped supply some protein. But I was biking thirty-five to fifty miles a day and chose routes with significant vertical climbs. So, I ate some pecorino cheese, yogurt, and eggs to help get some additional protein. Flexibility when you travel really helps.

One possible way to ease into a plant-based diet is to start as a flexitarian. The idea is to reduce your consumption of animal-based products. Maybe you can eat one to two dinners a week without chicken, beef, or fish. This is a good first step on the path to a plant-based diet.

My own journey began when a vegan physician friend invited me to dinner. The whole family looked so healthy and robust, but especially the two teenagers. They didn't simply exude great health—they were also good athletes and great students, winning soccer games and going to top-rated universities.

Duly impressed, I took the plunge. It was tough at first. One complication was that my wife, Diane, is a "meat and potatoes" person. She warned our children that if they did not eat animal meat their growth and development would be stunted. I was surrounded at dinners by rare cuts of steak, lamb chops, chicken, hamburgers, etc. Especially with the concerns that I had, as most of us do in the beginning, that I would not get enough protein, I would sneak little pieces of meat. I found red meat, in particular, gamey and greasy and realized that our appetite for meat is acquired.

If your experience is like mine, transforming from an animal protein-based diet to one built around plants may take a few years.

Don't expect to evolve and transition overnight.

One thing that will change is the vocabulary you use to explain your eating habits. At first, you might offer an embarrassed clarification to a friend who notices you skipped your traditional meat dish at lunch or dinner. "I'm trying to eat less red meat," you might say. With time, more confident and prouder, you'd say: "I'm eating less animal meat." Finally, you would announce unabashedly, "I'm following a plant-based or vegetarian diet."

After eating plant-based meals exclusively for a while, I started seeing the benefits to my health. My elevated cholesterol dipped to 150 total, with a bad or LDL cholesterol of 86. My triglycerides fell to within normal range.

Although I am naturally lean, I shed a few pounds too. For lots of people, the weight loss that comes with a plant-based diet is a big bonus. We are not used to seeing people without significant excess body fat in the United States. But that's how vegetarians look, if they are not also eating junk food, starches, and sweets. Without the animal fat in your diet you will see the extra pounds you are holding onto slip away. As one of my overweight best friends says of vegetarians, "They look like they could use a good meal!" But there is often truth to what loved ones say about us. You need to be careful that you don't lose too much weight, particularly lean muscle mass. You will need to increase your food consumption significantly on a plant-based diet to make sure that you get enough calories, especially as you increase your aerobic exercise.

In assessing weight and appearance, you also have to look at the underlying structure of the person. What did your body look like in high school? Were you tall and thin? How much did you weigh? Chances are that's what you'll look like again on a healthy, whole-foods, plant-based diet. But, don't fret, not all plant-based dieters look skinny. There are Olympic athletes and bodybuilders who are vegetarians. What do you think of the muscles of a big beautiful horse? They don't eat meat and get all the protein they need from plant foods.

BASICS OF NUTRITION

Now that I have driven home the importance of what you eat, I want you to be aware that *how much* you eat in different food categories is critical too. As you are likely aware, you have dietary requirements that relate to your body weight. In the sports nutrition world, we refer to the number of grams of a nutrient that you need to consume daily per kilogram of total body weight, and the calories you need daily per kilogram of lean body weight, which is your total weight minus the weight of body fat. Naturally, a 68-kilogram (150-pound) man needs far less protein than a 91-kilogram (200-pound) man, unless the 200-pound man is significantly overweight. And an overweight man should base his estimated daily calories on feeding his ideal weight or lean mass, not his current excessive weight.

To fully grasp the shifts in eating habits that are part of the Vail Method, a refresher on the basics of nutrients might be helpful. Macronutrients fall into three categories: carbohydrates, protein, and fat. When digested, any type of food breaks down into one or more of these categories. Vegetables are primarily carbohydrates with dietary fiber and a small amount of protein. Cooking oil is fat. Meat is primarily protein and fat. In terms of calories, a gram of carbohydrates carries 4 calories, a gram of protein the same, but a gram of fat has a whopping 9 calories. This is why fatty foods such as fried dishes and ice cream tend to pack on the pounds.

Carbohydrates can be simple or complex. Simple, or refined,

carbs are found in sugar, breads, or pasta. Complex carbs are found in vegetables and whole grains. The advantage to complex carbohydrates is that they have to be digested and broken down to produce sugar, so they raise your blood sugar more slowly. The rate at which carbs transform to sugar is known as the glycemic index (GI). For example, if glucose has a GI of 103, rice crackers come in at 87, a boiled potato 78, and white bread 75, compared with a sweet potato at 63 and boiled brown rice at 68. In the legume family, rich in carbohydrates as well as protein, chickpeas or garbanzo beans have a GI of 28. A raw apple has a GI of 36, a raw orange 43, and watermelon 76.[13]

If you are following a plant-based diet, ideally you will get only 5-10 percent of your calories from protein. This lower protein intake reduces your vulnerability to cancer. In addition, some studies also show that the fewer calories you consume, the better your chances of living longer. [14]

Twenty amino acids provide the building blocks of protein. Nine of them are "essential," which means that they cannot be made by our bodies: histidine, isoleucine, leucine, lysine, methionine, threonine, tryptophan, and valine. You have to get them from food or supplements.

Friends and family members are going to tell you that animal protein is not equivalent nutritionally to plant protein. They are well-intentioned but misinformed. In reality, plant foods contain the same amino acids.

Still, some of you may be worried that plants are not providing all the protein you need. If you eat a plant-food and whole-grain diet, you will get enough protein. You don't really need to take a protein supplement. But should you choose to do so, a recommendable one is a plant-based pea and rice protein supplement. One reason for mixing rice and pea protein is that rice is high in cysteine and methionine, but low in lysine; the reverse is true for pea protein. For those of us "numbers" people who track how many grams of protein we get in a day, this kind of supplement will help in the transition. You can be assured that at breakfast alone, you consumed fifteen to twenty grams of protein with the average supplement drink. But as you will see in the next chapter, my bowl of super fortified oatmeal rivals this amount of protein. Unfortunately, in our toxic world of contaminated foods, these powdered protein supplements, which are also used in packaged protein snack bars, have been found to be contaminated with heavy metals such as arsenic and lead.[15]

Some eating plans view carbohydrates as the enemy. In the Vail Method, the opposite is the case. Carbs will supply the vast majority of your calories. Since many of you have been told for a long time that carbs are bad, let me walk you through how many carbs and other nutrients you will need.

SPORTS NUTRITION

To calculate the optimal quantities of calories and nutrients you should be consuming daily in each category, you have to factor in your body weight—your fat-free mass—and your workout and activity levels. Different amounts of nutrients are required for jogging, racing, or other pursuits. See chapter 3 for an in-depth discussion of body fat measurements.

For energy consumption, the convention is to speak of calories consumed per kilogram of fat-free weight. To calculate your fat-free mass, we need to know your percentage of body fat. One pound of our body weight in the metric system equals 2.2 kilograms. So, first your weight in pounds is divided by 2.2 to get your weight in kilograms (kg). This number is multiplied by (100 – your percent body fat), then divided by 100. As an example, if we take 160 pounds and divide by 2.2 we get 72.72 kg. Now let's say you have 15 percent body fat. In that case, 100 – 15 percent body fat = 85, which divided by 100 is 0.85. We multiply 0.85 times 68 kilograms to get 61.81 kilograms of fat-free weight or FFM, fat-free mass. So, for your calorie allotment we would use 61.81 kilograms of fat-free weight to determine this.

The International Society of Sports Nutrition (ISSN) recommends consuming 25-35 calories per kilogram of fat-free body mass. This guideline applies to individuals engaging in moderate activity— exercise three times per week for thirty to forty minutes per session.[16] If you weigh 160 pounds with 15 percent body fat your allowance would be 2,163 calories per day. Someone who weighed 160 pounds with 20 percent body fat would be allotted only 2,036 calories, since we are not trying to nourish body fat.

Again, the calories per kilogram just noted is your body weight less your body fat, or your fat-free mass. If your workout activity is heavy, you will need more calories. The International Olympic Committee (IOC) advises a higher range—35-45 calories per kilogram of fat-free body mass per day.[17] This would take us up to 2,781 calories per day for the 160-pound, 15 percent body fat athlete, using the 45 calories per kilogram target. Some elite and Olympic athletes consume as much as 6,000 calories a day or higher.

Your caloric needs will vary on the days that you exercise versus your off days. You can make a reasonable assumption that if you are getting all the macronutrients in adequate amounts for your level of activity you will be consuming the proper number of calories. An easy metric to follow to determine if you are consuming the right number of calories is whether you are maintaining, losing, or gaining weight.

For carbohydrates and protein, the convention is to recommend grams of macro nutrient per kilogram of body weight rather than per fat-free mass. In some studies, you may see "ideal body weight" utilized. If someone exercises three times per week for thirty to forty minutes per session, the recommended range for daily carbohydrate consumption is 3-5 grams per kilogram of body weight. That comes to around 300 grams of carbs daily for an active 150-pound person.[18]

Timing of carbohydrate consumption is also important. Three factors determine optimal timing.[19] First, are you training or racing? For athletic performance, we speak of "carbohydrate loading" before exercise or a race to build your glycogen stores. Typically, this refers to carbohydrate consumption the night before a morning run or bike ride. It can also mean eating carbohydrates at least ninety minutes before the workout. If time allows, you can consume a more substantial meal three hours before a race to allow for digestion.

Second, occasionally we need to consume carbs during exercise. This is really only necessary for workouts lasting longer than an hour. In such cases, muscle fatigue and hypoglycemia are more likely as glycogen stores are depleted. These cause reactions that athletes call "hitting the wall" during the race, and slower recovery from exercise. For training workouts beyond an hour, you will need 30-60 grams of carbohydrates per hour, and for ultra-endurance races up to 90 grams per hour.[20] However, according to sports nutritionist Ryan Kohler at the CU Boulder Sports Medicine and Performance Center in Colorado, some well-trained recreational endurance athletes may need this supplementation for events lasting only one hour. This is true for those of us who have a high glycolytic capacity or metabolism, which we will discuss further in chapter 6. Athletes in this category burn a lot of sugar during aerobic activity and not as much fat as other recreational athletes. We are not attempting to compare any of the recreational athletes to the elite or professional athletes whose fat metabolism in endurance exercise is amazing—as you will see in chapter 6.

Carbohydrate consumption during a race typically involves a combination of gels, liquids, and some solids. A gel pack will have around 20 grams of carbohydrate. A sports drink such as Gatorade has 35 grams in twenty ounces.

There is a window of up to the first hour after exercise to maximize the replenishment of carbohydrates. You should be targeting 1.0-1.5 grams per kilogram of body weight. It is commonly preached in the sports world that the simultaneous consumption of protein helps with glycogen synthesis in the first thirty minutes post exercise. The protein would be approximately one gram for each three to four grams of carbohydrate consumed, or .2-.5 grams of protein per kilogram of body weight.[21] This suggested protein-to-carbohydrate ratio is primarily true when less than 1.0-1.5 grams per kg of carbohydrates are consumed, and not as big a concern when adequate carbohydrates in this range are eaten. Also, as our knowledge continues to grow by leaps and bounds, we're recognizing that the total consumption of calories, carbohydrates, and protein over the course of a day is more important than specific timing within the first hour after exercise.

Endurance exercise is known to increase oxidation, or utilization of leucine, one of the branched-chain amino acids (BCAA).[22] So, your protein source should include leucine as well as the other branched-chain amino acids involved in protein building, isoleucine and valine.

This eating program presents some interesting challenges, especially for vegans. Can you have sweet potatoes and black beans in a burrito shell available right after a workout—and is your stomach up to it? As an alternative, do you risk the heavy metal contaminants in a brown rice and pea protein supplement powder?

Few topics are as challenging to grasp scientifically as protein requirements, especially for athletes. And it's more complicated for someone on a plant-based diet.

Again, let's look at this in terms of grams of protein per kilogram of body weight. The Recommended Daily Allowance (RDA) of protein is 0.8 grams per kilogram of body weight. RDAs were initially developed in 1941 by the Food and Nutrition Board of the United States National Academy of Sciences.[23] RDAs include an amount considered adequate plus an added cushion, equal to the standard deviation, to avoid cutting anyone short on protein. If we go back to our 150-pound, or 68-kilogram person, that equals 54 grams of protein. Is that enough for someone doing really intense exercise?

Some sports nutrition specialists look at the person exercising three times a week for forty-five minutes and recommend consumption of 1.0 gram per kilogram. That's 68 grams of protein for a 150-pound person. For a vegan, that is going to be close to the maximum that can reasonably be consumed. It's the equivalent of about as many lentils, beans, and quinoa as a person can eat in a day.

Finally, some sport societies such as the American College of Sports Medicine recommend even higher levels of consumption for endurance athletes: 1.2-1.7 grams per kilogram per day.[24] The International Olympic Committee recommendation is 1.3-1.8 grams per kilogram for endurance athletes and 1.6-1.7 grams per kilogram for strength-training athletes.[25] As an example, 1.5 grams per kilogram for a 68-kilogram (150-pound) person would put your protein requirement at 102 grams per day. These studies focus more on building muscle than maintaining muscle mass.

Before leaving the topic of protein requirements I should mention the other side of the coin. Some authors who study societies with greater longevity have suggested protein consumption as low as 0.35 grams per kilogram is optimal for maximizing longevity. Similarly, some experts believe that consuming 100 grams of protein per day is way beyond what is necessary. Thus, the confusion in this area of nutrition is significant.

I am aware that the examples I use here of hard-driving athletes and their requirements do not apply to many of you. I mention them to give you a good yardstick to use in calculating your needs based on your level of activity. Again, in the Vail Method we encourage you to design a nutrition program that works for *you*. We are tracking your weight, body fat percentage, glycogen storage, maintenance of muscle mass, cholesterol, energy, and athletic performance, among other factors. While we trust the research studies that show a plant-based diet is best, we also want you to remember what your mother told you: do everything in moderation. For us, that means that as you follow a plant-based diet in pursuit of health benefits, you should not forget to live a little.

Life has so much to experience, including different people, places, and cultures. Let's say you're visiting Spain and your hosts offer you some wine and proudly boast of their Iberian ham. Should you not take a small taste? Why not! If you are in Maui and a wonderful fresh catch of fish is brought in, it won't kill you if you eat some. Some studies show that even with some occasional detours, the health benefits of a plant-based diet remain. In fact, in the Adventist Health Study 2, which followed 73,308 participants in Loma Linda, California, longevity was slightly higher among the vegetarians who included some fish in their diet versus the strict vegans, although the frequency of consumption was not clarified in the survey.[26]

I have gained an interesting perspective on life and aging by reading studies of populations that are notable for higher percentages of long-lived people. These communities are referred to as "Blue Zones" by *National Geographic* writer Dan Buettner.[27] People in these communities eat a diet built around vegetables, legumes, and plant-based foods. But they also include some fish and occasional meat. Longevity is attributed not just to the diet, but also the lifestyle that the people live (or once lived) in these special communities.

In Sardinia, Italy, as an example, the men who lived the longest were the shepherds who transported livestock from the mountains to the plains, often traveling for months at a time. Compared to hard-working farmers in other parts of Italy, these men were ten times as likely to live to one hundred.[28] A Sardinian diet in the 1930s included fava beans, barley, fennel, goat's milk, sheep's cheese, occasional meat, olive oil, tomatoes, eggplant and other vegetables, almonds, and wine. The islanders cooked with lard and ate fried eggs for breakfast. Protein content, overall, was low. But theirs was hardly a strict vegan diet.

I caution against comparing the circumstances in Blue Zones too closely to what goes on in our lives. We must consider the stress we endure daily and its effect on how we age. With frequent intrusions from smart phones, social media, work, and family matters, few of us live like wandering sheep herders. Genetics play an important role as well. In chapter 9, I explore the need for rest and relaxation as part of stress management.

Bottom line: don't close yourself off from interesting culinary experiences, and be more flexible when you're not eating at home. I am thinking of a young vegan woman who was trying a restaurant for the first time. The eatery served primarily classic American fare, but did make an excellent homemade veggie burger. She was intrigued, but asked about the bun. It was a soft bread and she worried whether it was vegan. Maybe it contained eggs or butter. She chose a salad instead. When my burger came, I offered her a taste of the burger without the bun. She smiled when she tasted it, because it was so good. See what I mean?

Maintain balance in your perspective. Dean Ornish, MD, was one of our early physician colleagues to demonstrate the reversal of heart disease with a plant-based diet. He has accomplished a remarkable achievement of having Medicare and private insurance carriers approve his "Intensive Cardiac Rehabilitation Program" for insurance coverage. He has, however, clarified his position for those seeking preventive dietary interventions. In *The Spectrum*, one of his later works, Ornish reiterated that a vegan diet is best, but added that those not currently suffering from heart disease have room for some flexibility. All individuals should try to find their place on that spectrum, a diet that works for them. That said, he has shown that there is a relationship between greater adherence to his lifestyle program and a more pronounced improvement in health, reversal of heart disease, and reduction of risk factors for chronic disease. His intensive cardiac rehabilitation program includes a whole-foods, plant-based, extremely low-fat diet as well as exercise, meditation, and a support group.

MAKING A LIFESTYLE CHANGE

In making a lifestyle change such as the Vail Method the potential results must outweigh the effect of any changes or sacrifices. You can ask yourself why some people continue to smoke when it's common knowledge that it's not good for us. The science is there and continues to mount each year about the benefits to your health of avoiding animal meats and eating a whole-foods plant-based diet. But will telling you this, or scaring you about getting diabetes and heart disease with the standard American diet, make you change, and stick to it? Or telling you that cultures of cancer cells were eight times more likely to die when exposed to blood from vegans?[29] Probably not. Maybe the increased chance to live longer will. What's more likely to convince you are the immediate positive results in your life. They are there for you in the Vail Method! Try it. You'll like it.

Obviously, it's easier if you already have a problem that needs attention. If you have chest pain from heart disease, and switching to this diet can give quick results, that's an easier incentive for you to remain devoted to the cause. But, do you need to get to the point of having chest pain when walking to stimulate you? Dr. Ornish has shown that participants in his intensive cardiac rehabilitation program have is an 84 percent reduction in chest pain in just two weeks, and 91 percent in 1 month![30] That's a home run, and therefore patients stick with his program.

Diet is an important part of my program, but there is much more to it, as you will see in later chapters on fitness, sleep, and meditation. Next, we will work on making this dietary transition practical for you.

CHAPTER FIVE

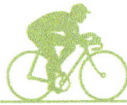

MAKING A PLANT-BASED DIET PRACTICAL FOR YOU

I have been preparing my own plant-based meals for several years and along the way I've picked up quite a few tips and techniques. I will show you some relatively easy ways to prepare plant-based dishes that you can eat for breakfast, lunch, and dinner. One thing I do not want to do here is create another cookbook filled with dishes that I like. Nor do I want to dictate a menu to you. What you eat is going to come down to what suits you best and what you like. I just want to give you some inspiration and a sense of how easy and fun it can be to plan and cook a plant-based bill of fare.

One adjustment many of you may have to make is in portion sizes. As I discussed in chapter 4, you need to consume certain levels of carbs and protein to fuel higher levels of exercise. For some, this will mean getting used to bigger portions than you might normally eat. I want to guide you in making those adjustments.

I also want to make you aware of certain foods you should avoid. And I'll point out the growing concerns about potential toxicity in some food products.

Getting used to a plant-based diet will take time and effort. Let it flow naturally. At times you will find yourself in situations where plant-based options are not easily available. I will talk about what to do in such cases.

Many people on plant-based diets prepare staples over the weekend to speed the process of making weekday meals. Please avoid the trap of relying on processed vegetarian meals in the grocery frozen foods section to save some time in the kitchen.

Under the Vail Method, you can eat healthier than that fairly easily. We want you to eat the original plants from nature, not processed foods with too many calories, sugar, and unhealthy oils. You'll lose excess weight by eating whole grains such as brown rice and quinoa with veggies, rather than white rice, pastas, or casseroles with cheese or fatty sauces. That's a big part of what the Vail Method is about.

Beans—an important source of plant protein—can be a great staple. Many people use canned beans. That's easy and fine. But the canned products don't compare in taste and texture to the freshly cooked ones—which typically require soaking and a few hours of cooking to prepare. This can be sped up significantly in a pressure cooker.

Beans come in many varieties. The US is the global leader in dry bean production, so access to just about any type is easy. Of course, dozens of brands of canned beans can work well in various recipes, too. But once you taste freshly prepared beans you will be spoiled.

Whole grains also lend themselves to advance preparation.

Quinoa is simple to cook and can be stored in the refrigerator for meals during the week. I've learned to make it easily in a rice cooker. It prepares quickly, so turn the cooker off when there is still a small layer of water in the bottom, to avoid it burning or sticking. The quinoa will cook the rest of the way. I use the same method for preparing brown rice. I discuss an alternative of boiling the brown rice and pouring off the excess water below. There are many varieties of grains that you can mix, such as millet, amaranth, and spelt. Some natural food stores and grocery sections carry mixtures of these grains.

Many vegans cook a large pot of steel-cut oatmeal over the weekend. You can enjoy a bowl with some cinnamon and walnuts. Then you can store the remaining oatmeal to reheat during the week. I'll give more details on other nutritional goodies you can add below, and the nutrition you will derive from a bowl of my super oatmeal.

Salads are hugely popular with plant-based diet devotees. Be creative in making them. Avoid the typical toss of iceberg lettuce or field greens, cucumber, and tomatoes. My version of a superfood salad starts with the freshest greens I can get. This usually is some red leaf lettuce coupled with chopped kale. Depending on the time of year, I might rely on packed field greens.

Then the fun begins. Add some carrots, chickpeas, and black beans. I like to sprinkle hemp seeds and chia seeds on for some healthy omega-3 fats and protein. Slice up some juicy tomatoes and top it all with a cup of quinoa. If you like the taste of ginger, you can add peeled and sliced fresh turmeric. It has great health benefits and is in the ginger family. I review the nutritional content of this superfood salad mix below.

Potatoes are another great source of carbohydrates and protein for your meals and easy to cook in the oven alongside other dishes or by themselves.

As I discussed in chapter 4, your body requires certain levels of nutrients. The amount of carbohydrates and proteins that works best varies for each person, according to his or her weight and level of physical activity on any given day. We reviewed caloric, protein, and carbohydrate requirements for someone following the Vail Method and exercising about three times a week for forty-five minutes. If you recall, the suggested amounts of protein vary significantly. At the low end are suggestions from experts in plant-based nutrition interested in maximizing the preventive health aspect of the diet; at the high end are guidelines from sports nutrition societies interested in growing muscle. This range goes from 0.8 to 1.7 grams of protein per kilogram of body weight. That's quite a spread and it's difficult to resolve and avoid confusion. I'm going to stick with a target of 0.8-1.0 grams per kilogram for a physically active person performing aerobic exercise at least three times per week, including some weight training. That's 54-68 grams of protein per day for a 150-pound person. The recommendation for carbohydrates would be approximately 300 grams a day for that same person.

MEETING YOUR NUTRITION GOALS ON A PLANT-BASED DIET: FOOD SOURCES AND PORTION SIZES

Four foods that I have found to be great ways to meet the protein requirements are chickpeas, quinoa, black beans, and lentils. Usually I cook one cup of dry quinoa in two cups of water. This produces four cups of cooked quinoa (see Figure 5.1).

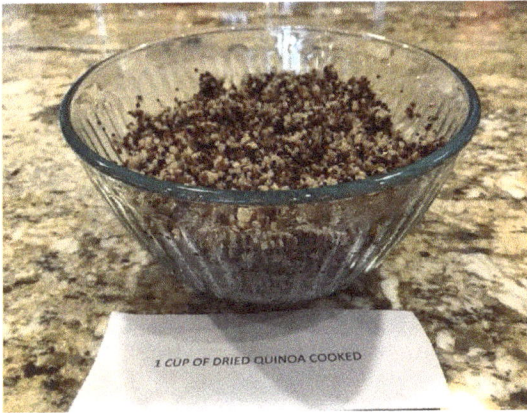

Figure 5.1: Four cups of cooked quinoa prepared from one cup of dry quinoa.

One cup of cooked quinoa (see Figure 5.2), a standard serving portion, contains 150 calories, 27 grams of carbs, 5 grams of protein, 3 grams of fiber, and 3 grams of fat. Quinoa is a complete protein source—in other words, it contains all the essential amino acids.

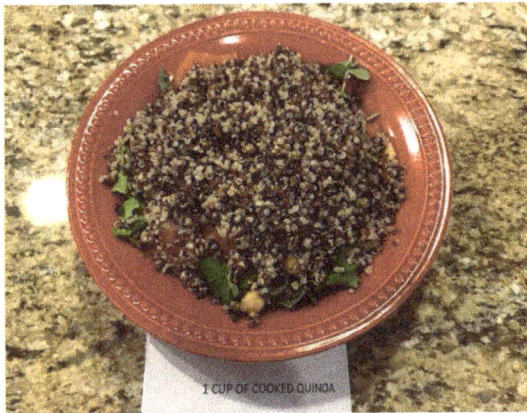

Figure 5.2: One cup of cooked quinoa atop a mixed green salad.

What I would like to illustrate in Figure 5.2 is how a cup of quinoa looks in a salad. Pay attention to restaurant salads with quinoa in the name, and realize how little you normally get.

I use a similar approach in cooking chickpeas and black beans. I start with a cup of dried beans and soak them in water overnight on Saturday. The prep work only takes a minute. Pour the beans into a pot half filled with water. On Sunday, bring the beans to a boil and then simmer them for two hours or so, depending on the bean type and how soft you like them to be.

Once cooked, a cup of dried chickpeas yields around four cups or four servings. Each one-cup serving (Figure 5.3) constitutes around 250 calories, 9 grams of protein, 9 grams of fiber, and 30 grams of carbohydrates. The process of preparing black beans is similar.

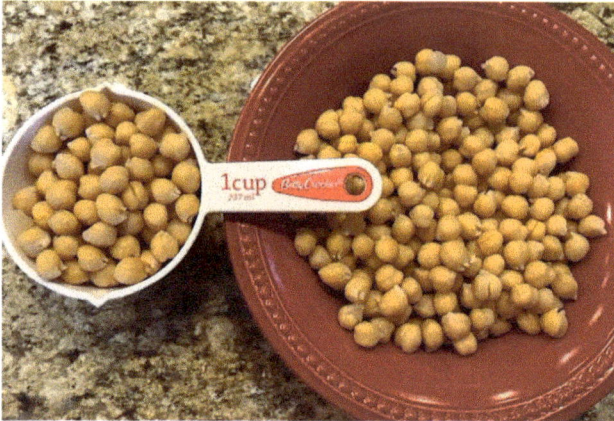

Figure 5.3: One cup of cooked chickpeas.

As you can see, this is a lot of chickpeas to eat in a salad. Also note this is 9 grams of protein. So, if you throw just a handful of garbanzos in a salad, how much protein are you getting? Not much. You need to be mindful of what you are consuming.

I usually add half a cup of chickpeas and half a cup of black beans to my salads. Notice in Figure 5.4 the difference a half- cup serving makes.

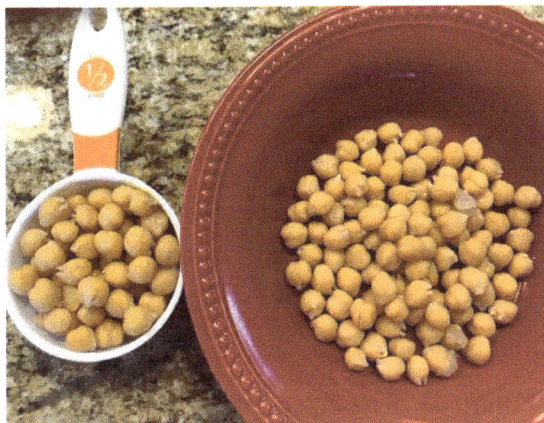

Figure 5.4: Half-cup serving of cooked chickpeas

This is still a lot more beans than many of you are used to, but I find it easier to mix up a variety of beans and legumes to hit some protein, carbohydrate, and calorie targets.

THE SUPERFOOD SUPER SALAD

For those of you keeping track, the half cup of cooked garbanzo beans or chickpeas and the half cup of cooked black beans combined yield 9 grams of protein, 30 grams of carbs, and 250 calories. Don't forget to add the one cup of cooked quinoa for another 5 grams of protein, 27 grams of carbs, and 150 calories. So, we are at 14 grams of protein, 57grams of carbs, and 400 calories. I also sprinkle about a tablespoon of organic hemp hearts, or shelled hemp seeds, into the salad. That adds another 3 grams of protein and 4 grams of omega-3 and -6 fatty acids and about another 60 calories. I also add a table-spoon of chia seeds with another 50 calories and 2 grams of protein. These seeds add some healthy fats that contribute to my caloric needs as a distance runner. This salad alone will not cut it for runners doing significant distances. But for you protein counters, this salad is at

19 grams. However, in working with patients, I find these servings provide way more beans then they are accustomed to eating. That's why I'm showing you some photos of portion sizes.

One other tip on the Superfood super salad. My family jokes about how long it takes me to mix a variety of lettuce and kale leaves and rinse and strain them, wash and slice tomatoes, sprinkle in the seeds described above, add the garbanzo and black beans, and finally the large cup of quinoa. I also grate fresh turmeric when available, and slice fresh carrots. So, my solution has been to prepare three salads at a time, to cover the next three days.

Many of you will be pioneers in your family in your commitment to a healthier plant-based diet. Like any worthwhile challenge faced by trailblazers, this is not an easy path to forge. You may deal with verbal assaults about vegetarians and comments about how restrictive and boring a non-meat-based diet is.

If you are not the primary cook in the family, your challenges are greater. Whoever has that role will be asked to prepare two types of meals when one was challenging enough with his or her other responsibilities. Or you will need to prepare your own.

A few tips apply here. As you eliminate meat, look to replace it with plant-based foods that are rich in protein.

Legumes are a natural choice, and an easy way to prepare them involves a process known as "sprouting." It involves allowing lentils, mung beans, or quinoa to sprout with water and air until the beginning of a new plant takes form. This breaks down the hard, outer protective shell of the lentil, mung bean, or quinoa and allows for quicker cooking and more release of nutrients. These sprouted legumes are then dried and packaged for the grocery shelf. You can readily find them in many supermarkets or at a natural grocer. You simply add a quarter-cup of sprouted product to water that is boiling in a small pot. In approximately four minutes, depending on your preference for the degree of softness, you have a healthy addition to any meal. Use a strainer to pour out the water, and you are ready to eat. Let's say you are having soup with dinner. You can easily add sprouted lentils to your bowl, or simply eat them as a side dish on your plate. A quarter-cup serving of sprouted lentils, for example, has a whopping 9 grams of protein, and the great news is that it is a relatively small and manageable amount to consume (See Figure 5.5).

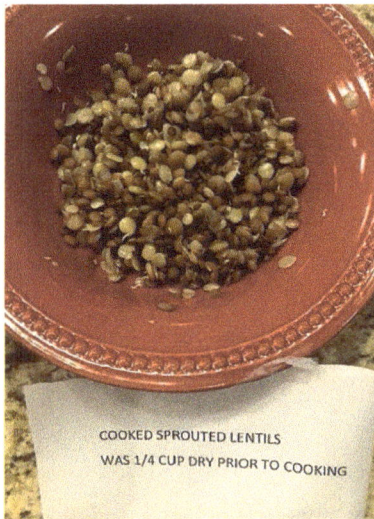

COOKED SPROUTED LENTILS
WAS 1/4 CUP DRY PRIOR TO COOKING

Figure 5.5: cooked sprouted lentils from a quarter-cup dry serving.

Soy is another excellent protein source. A popular way to consume it is edamame. Frozen organic edamame is widely available and easy to prepare. All you need to do is put the pods in a vegetable steamer and defrost for a few minutes. Sprinkle them with salt and watch them disappear. One and one-eighth cup of edamame in the pod will yield a half-cup of shelled edamame, which contains 8.5 grams of protein.

THE MORNING BOWL OF OATMEAL

I've beefed up (yikes, that's a poor choice of words) my morning bowl of oatmeal. The basic ingredient is a half-cup dry weight serving of steel-cut oatmeal cooked in water. This has 150 calories, 27 grams of carbs, 3 grams of fiber, 2.5 grams of fat, and 4 grams of protein. Quick-cooking oats prepared in the microwave yield different numbers for a serving: a half cup dry contains 180 calories, 29 grams of carbs, and 7 grams of protein. Prior to cooking it in the microwave, I add 1.5 tablespoons of ground organic flaxseeds. A serving of flaxseeds can be listed as whole or ground seeds. I freshly grind my seeds once a week for better absorption. In my Vitamix blender, two tablespoons of whole seeds yield three tablespoons when ground. Figures 5.6 and 5.7 help clarify serving sizes.

A tablespoon and a half of ground flaxseeds has about 60 calories, with 2 grams of omega-3 fatty acids (alpha linoleic acid), 2.5 grams of fiber, 4 grams of carbohydrates, and 2.5 grams of protein.

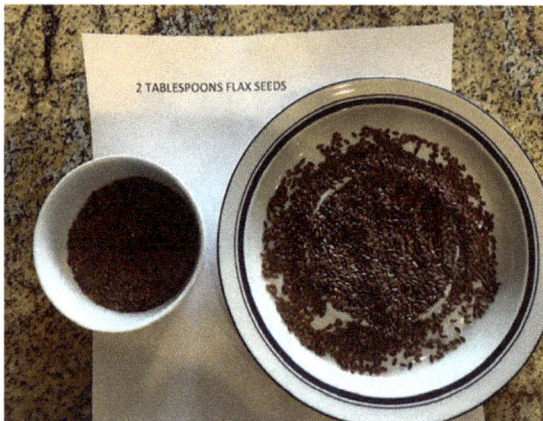

Figure 5.6: Two tablespoons whole flax seeds

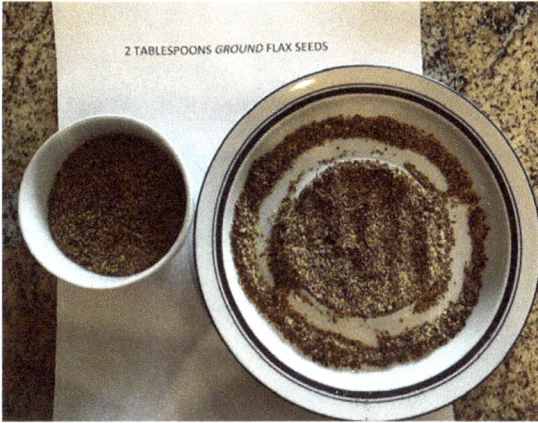

Figure 5.7: Two tablespoons ground flax seeds.

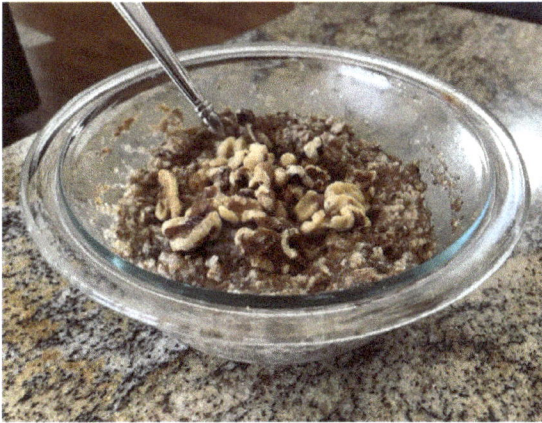

Figure 5.8: Souped-up oatmeal.

To this dry mix of oatmeal and ground flax, I add one tablespoon of Kretschmer wheat germ, which adds 30 additional calories, 4 grams of carbohydrates, and 2 grams of protein. I then add a sprinkle of cinnamon and touch of brown sugar. After the oatmeal is cooked and stirred, I top it with a quarter cup of walnuts, which has 190 calories, 18 grams of fat, 4 grams of carbohydrates, 2 grams of fiber, and 4 grams of protein (see Figure 5.8).

For numbers-oriented people, the total varies between the slow-cooked steel-cut oats and the quick-cooking oats. It ranges between 430 and 460 calories, 39-41 grams of carbohydrates, 8 grams of fiber, 12.5-15.5 grams of protein, and lots of healthy omega-3 and -6 fatty acids.

Another option is to add 1 tablespoon of chia seeds and 1 tablespoon of hemp hearts. This provides 120 calories, 5 grams of fiber, more healthy omega 3 and 6 fatty acids, and 6 grams of protein.

One final tweak is to add some unsweetened soy milk at the end. This does add some extra nutrition. A full 8 ounces has 80 calories, three grams of carbs, and seven grams of protein, but you'll use a fraction of this.

THE MOST RESTRICTIVE PLANT-BASED DIET

Some people with severe heart disease who are attempting to reverse the narrowing in the arteries of their hearts follow the most extreme version of this diet. They avoid all dairy products and eggs and limit fats as well. The small scoop of walnuts described for the oatmeal would be a full day's allowance of saturated fat for them, and some would even frown upon this. They avoid cooking oils and avocado as well.

My position is that limiting fat this severely is not necessary for those eating a plant-based diet to avoid or prevent cardiac disease. Others disagree, and believe in preaching this vegan, no-fat diet to all. From a public health standpoint, we stand a better chance of improving the health of millions through less-restrictive whole-food plant-based diets, especially if they can replace habits like consuming animal protein, minimal vegetables, insufficient fiber, etc.

As you get more comfortable with a plant-based diet, be aware of the foods you should sidestep. There's a food revolution going on. The diet we espouse in the Vail Method is riding the crest of that wave. We're learning that what we've been fed as truth by biased groups representing the dairy and meat industries is in fact misinformation. You don't need massive amounts of protein and it doesn't have to come from animals. A plant-based diet will not stymie your athletic pursuits.

Rich Roll showed us that the sky can be the limit in terms of athletic achievement for those of us on plant-based diets. You may be familiar with Roll's story, told in his book, *Finding Ultra*. He transformed himself from a life of alcohol overconsumption into a vegan athlete who runs ultramarathons. In a different biography, *Eat and Run: My Unlikely Journey to Ultramarathon Greatness*, Scott Jurek shared how he embraced a vegan diet that powers him through one-hundred-mile races.

One thing you should limit is your consumption of dairy. Try to reduce cow's milk (and other animal milk) in your diet. One of the major concerns is the elevated hormone content of cow's milk.[31] Reliable studies have demonstrated the increased risk of cancers that respond to sex hormones, such as prostate cancer.[32] An increased incidence of Parkinson's disease among dairy consumers is another issue.[33] In addition, high levels of pesticides in dairy are troubling to some.[34]

I would like to add some balance and perspective to these studies about dairy consumption and increased risk of cancer and Parkinson's disease. As I read through them the findings and conclusions are not as simple and straightforward as one would like them to be. For example, some studies found associations only with low-fat dairy such as skim milk, but not whole milk,[35] and some studies found minimal or no association. The more dairy consumed in these studies, however, the higher the risk for prostate cancer and Parkinson's disease.

My point is that the old adage "everything in moderation" holds some weight here. If you want to reduce your risk, avoid dairy products. But if you primarily use alternatives to milk as discussed below, and you still enjoy a traditional crema in your cappuccino, or a scoop of gelato when you visit Italy, how much risk are you adding?

Fortunately, there are many tasty alternatives to dairy. The objective is to get used to the taste of one of the healthier options. Almond milk works well in cereal as a dairy alternative. It's low in fat—only 2.5 grams in eight ounces. Soy milk is another popular choice with 7 grams of protein per cup. Coconut milk is not as good an option as it contains significant saturated fat. It's often found in dairy-free ice creams.

Sugar, in all of its forms, should also be avoided. That means not only pure sugar but also corn syrup, contained in many packaged foods. Sugar is found in most commercial cereals, breads, and processed carbohydrate products. Avoiding such foods is important because sugar stimulates the release of insulin, which forces the sugar out of your blood, into your cells, which in turn leads to a sugar low. Your body responds to the lower glucose level with weakness and food cravings. That explains why many people reach for a midmorning muffin, donut, or bagel.

Whenever possible, stick to complex carbohydrates with lower glycemic indexes. as discussed in chapter 4. Whole-grain brown rice is better than white rice, pasta, or bread. But you are actually better off filling your belly with wholesome vegetables. It's a learned habit. Even my teenaged kids have learned to gorge on steamed kale and broccoli, despite all the normal dietary fickleness that comes with being a teenager.

Try to lower the amount of added sugar in your diet. If you can't drink coffee without more than one sugar packet, try switching to green tea without sugar to get your morning caffeine. As you wean yourself away from sugar, you'll consume less and be better off.

In medicine, we refer to the downregulation of receptors. What does this mean? Our taste buds get used to high levels of sugar, and we automatically dump two or more teaspoons of it in our coffee. As you eat less processed sugar, you will find that you need to add less sugar to everything. So, your receptors or taste buds will respond favorably to lower levels of stimulation, or less sugar.

Once you get in the habit of eating the kinds of meals I describe here—and other healthy whole plant-based foods—you should get nearly all the nutrients you need. The only vitamin you will need is B12, an easy supplement to add to your regimen.

THE TOXIC WORLD OF FOOD: THE CHALLENGE FOR THE TWENTY-FIRST CENTURY

Some plant foods may include heavier doses of toxins. We live in a polluted, toxic world. Eating a plant-based diet will help reduce your carbon footprint—but it won't eliminate your exposure to known and unknown carcinogens. Regardless of whether you are a plant eater or a meat eater, one of the big challenges and problems of this century will be ongoing discoveries of the toxic effects that polluted oceans, soils, and water have on important food sources.

For years in integrative medicine we talked about the benefits of green tea, the best tasting of which comes from China. But we did not know until recently that the tea contained lead.[36] How did that happen? Chinese gas stations continued to provide leaded fuel long after it was banned in the US. The lead ended up in the soil, and thereby the roots of the tea plants. So, green tea from China is contaminated with lead. Is it a problem for green tea drinkers? Probably not. But should we limit the number of cups of tea in a day? Probably. Again, the wisdom of everything in moderation—whether it's growth stocks in your stock portfolio, or cups of green tea in a day—has merit.

Another toxin alert: arsenic in rice.[37] What could be better than some brown rice with our veggies? The answer is a bit complicated. Brown rice is grown in soil contaminated with pesticides containing arsenic. So white rice, the "bad" stuff with a higher glycemic index, may be safer for you in moderate amounts. Researchers have found one way to address the potential arsenic problem in brown rice: prepare it like pasta, boiling it in a large volume of water, then pour out the water.[38]

Brown rice protein concentrate, which is used in plant protein supplements, can also be a problem. Does the concentrate contain even higher levels of arsenic? We are told that the arsenic is highest in the outer shell of the rice, thus higher in brown rice than in white rice. But in producing brown rice protein concentrate, the outer shell reportedly is excluded. Enzymes are used that separate the carbohydrate part of the brown rice from the protein to create the concentrate.

• • •

With time, maintaining a plant-based diet at home will become second nature. Eating out in restaurants or at friends' homes, on the other hand, may pose more challenges.

Salads and bowls with quinoa are appearing on menus at some better fast-casual restaurants. But sadly, most fine-dining restaurants have yet to embrace plant-based menus other than superficially. Most restaurants consider a vegetarian option to be anything without meat. But they have little knowledge about plant-based proteins from beans and legumes. You'll be lucky if tofu is offered. Quinoa or other grains might be added to a salad, but often there is not enough to provide the protein and carbs your body needs.

You have to recognize that restaurants are a business and they need to appeal to the majority of guests to remain profitable. That means serving mostly meat dishes. That's what several chefs and restaurant owners have told me, even those who are aware of plant-based diets and their advantages.

If you have the opportunity to explore plant-based meals prepared at a great vegetarian restaurant, go for it! You will enjoy the variety of flavor and product available. At one such restaurant, even my meat-and-potatoes friend said to me, "I could eat this every day if someone prepared it for me."

Dining out—whether in restaurants or at homes of friends and family members—is where those of us devoted to a plant-based diet have to be more flexible. Sadly, I have seen friends limit dining-out occasions with other friends because they worry that the limited options in restaurants will not fit their diet. If you end up isolating yourself socially to follow this diet to the extreme, you may be doing more harm to your health than the occasional "chegan" or "cheating vegan" meal. We are social creatures and need to share meals as a means of interacting. Don't restrict or avoid this important part of your life.

In restaurants, you can and should be smart about ordering. On many menus, staples such as beans or kale that fit into the Vail Method diet may be offered as side dishes. If you encounter them on a menu, don't be shy about ordering double portions. While others may consider such dishes as afterthoughts, you might end up building your whole meal around them.

CHAPTER SIX

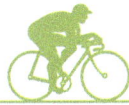

OPTIMIZING YOUR FITNESS ROUTINE, NO MATTER YOUR SPORT

We are now ready to explore how you can elevate your current aerobic capacity and athletic performance to create a better, stronger you—what we like to call your version 2.0. We have already discussed the tests you should undergo to determine your fitness level and capacity for more exercise. We're going to use the data from those tests to improve your fitness and help you set and reach higher goals.

For some that may mean better 10K, marathon, or bike racing times. If you're clocking in at three and a half hours in a marathon, for example, it could mean knocking twenty minutes or more off your time. For others, it may translate to improved health, fitness, and energy. Exercise physiology has come a long way. There is no question that if you follow the principles of the Vail Method, we can get you to the next level and beyond. This applies to everyone, from recreational fitness buffs and weekend warriors to elite athletes, from young to old alike.

Stepping up your fitness game involves many factors. I will try to cover the main categories here. For starters, I want to show you the ways we use your lactate threshold test results to calibrate a plan for your aerobic workouts. I will discuss some exercises for runners and bikers that can help strengthen muscles that are key to your sport. And I will also talk about what to do when you incur injuries or other stresses on the body.

In chapter 3, I described the lactate threshold test in detail. Now I'll walk you through why it was worth it to go through the huffing and puffing it entailed.

The examiner who performs the test should give you a graph of your lactate metabolism curve. Figure 6.1 is a chart of my first test in 2013 by Inigo San Millan, PhD, formerly of the UC Sports Medicine and Performance Center. If you recall, the Y axis on the left side of the graph shows my heart rate; the X axis shows the speed of the treadmill, which increases in five-minute intervals; and the Y axis on the right side shows my blood lactate level. Some key markers on the graph are what we call the inflection points—the points on the curve where your lactate levels (red line) jump as your heart rate (blue line) rises. We use these critical points to determine your heart rate range for exercise. (We'll cover that later in the chapter.)

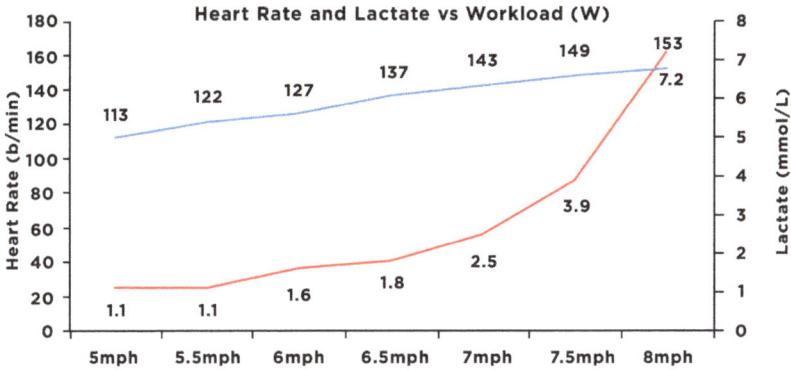

Figure 6.1: Heart rate and blood lactate level.

You also should receive another graph that shows your fat versus carbohydrate metabolism (see Figure 6.2). On my own graph you can see the fat and carbohydrate oxidation rates. The X axis is my heart rate. The left Y axis shows the rate at which I am burning carbohydrates (blue line). The right Y axis shows the fat consumption rate (red line). Also, note that at lower heart rates—particularly between 113 and 127—more fat is being burned. As exercise intensity and heart rate increase, fat burning drops significantly, and carbohydrate consumption continues to climb. We are looking at your heart rate to see where fat utilization peaks and where it begins to drop, as carbohydrate metabolism rises. This curve has an inflection point as well at around a heart rate of 122. We examine this graph along with the lactate curve.

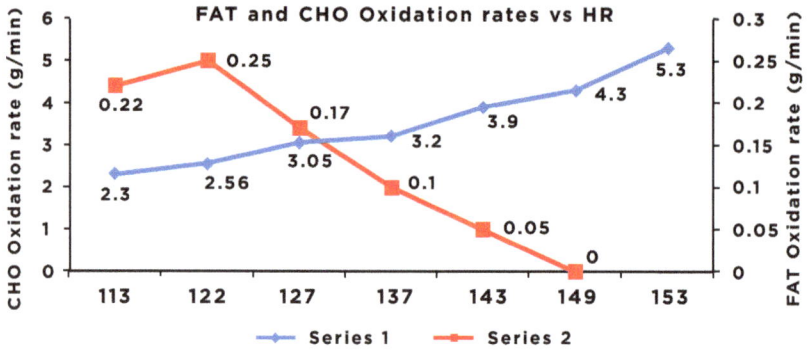

Figure 6.2: Carbohydrate and fat metabolism as a function of heart rate, according to methodology by Inigo San-Millan and George A. Brooks, "Assessment of Metabolic Flexibility by Means of Measuring Blood Lactate, Fat, and Carbohydrate Oxidation Responses to Exercise in Professional Endurance Athletes and Less-Fit Individuals," Sports Medicine 48, no. 2 (June 2017): 467, https://doi.org/10.1007/s40279-017-0751-x.

We can see the heart rate at which you begin to transition out of this key aerobic zone, when you are burning more fat than carbohydrate. An elite endurance athlete would still be burning fat at higher heart rates and work outputs as shown in Figure 6.3.

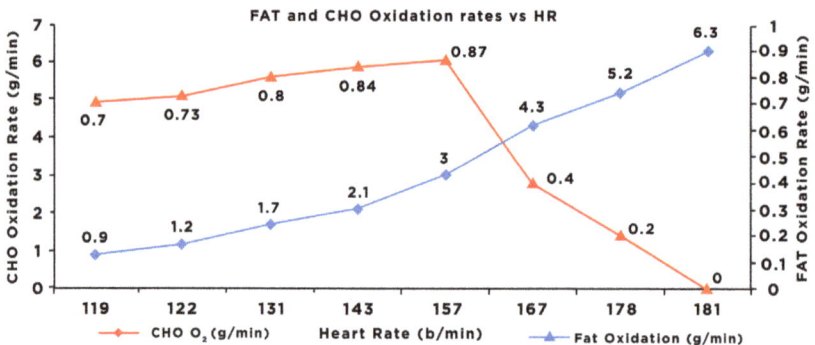

Figure 6.3: FAT and CHO oxidation rates versus heart rate for an elite athlete. Data provided by Inigo San Millan, PhD.

Note that our pro cyclist burns .87 grams of fat per minute, peaking at a heart rate of 160, compared to my peak fat metabolism of only .25 grams of fat, at about 124 beats per minute. Any question who would win an endurance race? Think of his work load, speed, and output while only coasting on his fat stores. In chapter 4, I spoke of athletes with a more glycolytic metabolism requiring more carbohydrate replacement during runs of one hour or longer. You can now understand that these athletes burn more carbohydrate than fat, at less exertional heart rates than others who are still burning fats. I do notice a difference when I replace carbs during a longer run.

You need to be burning fat for effective endurance training. Your glycogen stores will be depleted after about forty-five minutes of running or biking, and the remaining workout fuel can only come from fat—or from protein consumed from muscle, which is undesirable. With increasing exercise effort—think of faster speeds on a treadmill or a track—the amount of lactate that needs to be cleared is increasing as well. As you reach a certain level, which is specific to you at this phase in your training, the mitochondria begin to be overwhelmed by the amount of lactate that they need to process. Your blood lactate level rises. If it gets high enough, you will run out of energy, and the workout or race is over.

These graphs suggest the heart rate zone where you should be putting most of your training effort to build more and larger mitochondria, which are capable of allowing you to run or bike harder in a race when you need to, and still be able to use your long-lasting fat stores for fuel. As your lactate metabolism improves with training, you can run faster with higher heart rates than before, while still running your engine in a lower gear, because your engine is more powerful with bigger and more plentiful mitochondria. That is what we are doing: giving you more performance and power from a gear that burns less fuel than the one you've been using to get the same output from your engine.

AGELESS FITNESS

Before showing you how we derive a training program for you, I want to motivate you with some hard data from the physiology lab supporting your ability to "keep hammering it" at any age.

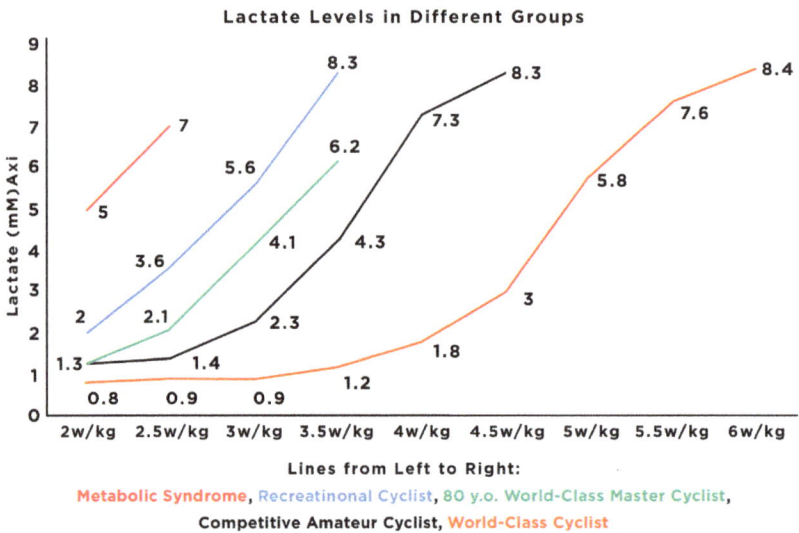

Figure 6.4: Lactate Threshold Testing on Cyclists. Data from Inigo San Millan, PhD

For Figure 6.4 above, our X axis is the power output of the cyclist in watts of energy per kilogram of their body weight. The higher the number, the harder they are working and the greater the amount of energy they are exerting. This would be the equivalent of speeding up the treadmill for our runners as we proceed to the right along the X axis.

The Y axis is the blood lactate level of the athlete. Remember that normal blood levels at rest are around 1.0 and rise with progressive exercise output. Also, lower lactate levels of 2.5 or less can be maintained for hours, as in a running marathon.

Figure 6.4 on the previous page, courtesy of Inigo San Millan, PhD, shows the lactate curves of five different cyclists from the left side of the graph to the right. On the far left is patient with the "metabolic syndrome." This is a situation unfortunately seen far too often in the United States and includes increased body fat, high blood sugar, high blood pressure, and elevated cholesterol. This "syndrome" places people at increased risk of a heart attack or developing diabetes. Note that at the low level of 2 watts of energy per kilogram exerted on the bicycle, their lactate level is already at 5.0!

Our second cyclist is a 40 year old who uses the bicycle for recreation and wellness but not a competitive cyclist. He clearly outperforms the person with the metabolic syndrome, as the lactate curves improve as we move to the right in the graph. Our third cyclist and third line to the right is an 80 year old master cyclist! Yes, I did say "eighty," and he still competes. He actually outperforms our 40 year old recreational cyclist. The lesson here is that age is not a barrier, at least until age 80, if training is done correctly as we preach.

The last two curves to the right, are for serious competitive cyclists. The fourth curve for an amateur competitive cyclist, and the last curve to the right for one of our pro cyclists.

I think that this graph, once understood, should inspire us all!

HOW DO WE DESIGN A HEART RATE BASED TRAINING PROGRAM?

The lactate graphs shown in figures 6.1 and 6.2 give us insight to optimize your training program.

Figure 6.1 shows the various exercise heart rate zones.

Zone 1, a heart rate under 128, corresponds to easy training. As seen in Figure 6.2, fat consumption is highest in this heart rate zone. The muscle fibers working at this level of exercise are the type I, slow twitch type.

Zone 2 is our targeted endurance heart rate, from 128 to 135. Fuel consumption in this zone is fat and carbohydrate. But fat consumption is dropping, and carbohydrate consumption is rising to where the two curves cross in Figure 6.2. Type I slow twitch fibers are still in use. This is the zone where you want to do most of your cardio work. This is where you will build your endurance and cardiac health the most. It is how you upgrade to a stronger engine.

Zone 3 should be reached during some of the intervals of your cardio work, and ranges in this example from heart rates of 136-146. This range uses some type IIa fast twitch, glycogen-fueled muscle fibers as well as type I.

Zone 4 is the lactate threshold. In this example, it ranges from a heart rate of 147- 152. This is the level at which the fuel source is all carbohydrates, which will be depleted quickly. Type IIa fast twitch muscle fibers are at work here.

Zones 5 and 6 take us above the lactate threshold into anaerobic metabolism. Lactate accumulation will quickly impede the athlete's performance. Muscles are burning and yearning to stop. Heart rates above 153, in this illustrated example, exceed this lactate threshold. For younger athletes, this anaerobic heart rate would be much higher.

Zone 5 would be used during a quick push in a race, a short accelera-tion of your engine when needed.

Most elite athletes devote the majority of their time—around eighty percent—to training at the lower heart rates, or zone 2. This is where they build their long-range potential. The same will hold true for your regimen. Your own test results will show your ideal heart rate target for training in zone 2. The same graph and technology apply, whether you are a weekend warrior or an elite athlete, and reveal the best heart rate for zones 3-5, the levels where you should be doing interval work. You need this to develop your higher-speed muscles for racing and when you need to push yourself.

I cite my case study here to give you a sense of how the test results are charted and used. Your plan will be based on your unique results.

When I first took the test in 2013, Dr. San Millan designed a training schedule to maximize my own potential. I train three times a week at the zone 2 level. Some of these sessions included interval work in zones 3-5. Sometimes, I'll do a shorter run of thirty minutes and mix in some seven-minute or longer high-intensity intervals, particularly when I'm doing my track work before a race. The goal: to improve my metabolic efficiency and lactate clearance capacity.

BUILDING FOR THE LONG RUN

When I repeated the test in 2018, my lactate tolerance levels had not changed much. It was great that I hadn't deteriorated in five years and held my own. But I hadn't improved either. So, Dr. San Millan revised my training regime a bit. To "move the needle" on my lactate test results, he asked me to run longer sessions, over an hour, rather than forty-five or fifty minutes. Or to go for longer, easier road bike rides, not as steep or as short in duration as my challenging rides on roads that go up alongside the ski mountains. So, I increased sixty minutes of cycling to ninety to 120 minutes and my runs to sixty to ninety minutes.

Most of you who are used to training for half or full marathons know that one run each week will be your "long run." I really noticed a difference in my ability to run much longer and bike much longer with slower, easier work, staying in a lower heart rate for my range of zone 2. This helped me immensely in preparing for the half marathon. The goal for everyone is to shift your curve in the direction of elite athletes, but you won't match their curve, of course, unless you decide to turn pro and put in the required time. By shifting the curve, I mean that you will be able to work out at higher intensity levels while still maintaining lower lactate levels that enable you to perform longer.

If your blood lactate level at rest is 1.0, you can run at a speed that builds your lactate level up to 2.0, and you could maintain this for hours. But if you sped up to a level that increases your lactate level to 4.0, you might only last forty-five to sixty minutes. That's why marathoners need to run at a low lactate level, usually around 2.5.

Just to summarize: there are two main components to shifting the curve. The first, as I've explained above, is working out at the heart rates that enhance your mitochondrial function and reach your goal. The second is following a training program that specifies the optimal frequency and duration of each session to achieve this effect. Following a consistent diet with adequate calories and carbohydrates to fuel your body is essential, as is getting adequate sleep and following the other parts of the Vail Method.

Once you start to get into the rhythm of your regime, one thing I recommend apart from regular, consistent training is that you participate in races or other organized events. Most big races offer walks as well. The only one you are competing with is yourself, to see how well you can do. How did your time compare with your last outing?

There are a couple of reasons this is a good idea. One is to give you a goal to work toward. Can you build to a half marathon, marathon, or ultra-endurance event? If you're a walker now, can you go six miles, or run? The other reason is to feel the excitement of the start gun going off and running like a pack of gazelles. It's great to experience the movement of so many athletes with you.

There are always going to be many people faster than you, so don't worry about them, or how your pace compares to theirs, and don't make a beginner's mistake of trying to run too fast and chase them. You've only prepared for *your* race, whatever your pace is at this point. You now understand that while others appear to be flying by, their superior engines are only running at a lower lactate level. Chasing them would just raise your lactate too high, and you would burn out. You will get to higher highs if you like. That's the plan. Just be patient and hang in there. When you walk to the start line, you should know what your race pace and finish time should be.

Each year on Memorial Day, I run the Bolder Boulder in Colorado with fifty thousand like-minded individuals. Runners start in groups of about a thousand, with groups spaced a minute apart. Your group is determined by your pace last year, or in another sanctioned ten-kilometer run. My goal each year is to see if I can stay in the same group. So far, after twelve years, I have succeeded, or dropped a level, only to regain it the next year. As I mentioned earlier, I took fifth for my age in the 2018 race, which was nice, but it was holding my pace and time that pleased me the most.

INJURY PREVENTION

No matter what your preferred sport, the more you step up your training game, the more susceptible you are to strains on the body. For aerobic athletes who pursue this as a way of life, the loss of an activity we are passionate about, even a temporary break, is a threat.

You should take every precaution to stave off injury. One thing I do and recommend is resting a day between hard workouts to allow minor strains and pains to recover. I've achieved very competitive race times with this approach and enjoyed decades of injury-free running. If you want to run five days or more per week, at least plan for some easy days, or alternate with resistance weight training in the gym.

I am also a big advocate of stretching. Many injuries occur after failure to stretch followed by exertion. After a long night's sleep, we are stiff. Think of the marvelous creatures in our animal kingdom. How many times a day does your cat stretch on getting up from a nap before jumping up on the counter? As significant as stretching is preceding exercise, it is also important to stretch your muscles after a good workout.

In stretching, we want to focus on specific areas for different sports. For example, runners get tight hip flexors, hamstrings, and Achilles tendons. You should also incorporate spine extension, or bending backward, into your stretching routines, especially if you have lower back pain or lumbar disc problems.

To inspire you, I'll mention a couple of stretches here. For your Achilles tendon, all runners know how to lean on the wall with both arms straight in front of them. The right leg is bent at the knee, and the left leg is kept straight and far behind the right. This of course stretches the left Achilles. The more that the left leg is slid back, further behind the right, the greater the stretch.

One excellent stretch involves lying on your back on a mat, bending your right knee up to your chest, and placing a long rope around the sole of that foot. Now pull the rope up toward the sky to straighten that leg. This provides a great hamstring stretch and is safer than trying to bend from your waist. Do both sides, of course. For runners, after you straighten the leg toward the sky, pull the rope across your body to stretch your iliotibial or "IT" band.

Two yoga poses—the downward dog and upward dog—are excellent ways to stretch the back of your legs and your spine. The spine is a crucial part of the body that many athletes fail to protect. Most lower spine injuries, herniated discs, or sciatica come from excessive flexion of our spines. We need to work on extending our spines to offset the excessive movements we make in flexion.

The easiest and most useful of the spine stretches I do is one my teen-aged son refers to as "girlie pushups." Here you lie flat on a mat, face down, belly touching the mat, legs extended straight behind you. Next you place your hands on the floor, in what looks like the preparation for a pushup. Instead, you keep your waist and belly button in contact with the floor, and slowly push up with your arms to raise your head and back. Come down slowly and repeat again, this time ideally extending your spine more, and rising higher.

Another favorite, for stretching your quadriceps muscles, is lying on your side, grasping your lower leg around the ankle, and bending your lower leg up toward your back.

To stretch your piriformis muscle and gluteals, you can do the following exercise one of two ways. Lying flat on a mat, raise both legs off the ground, then cross your right leg over the left, such that your right foot and ankle rest on your left knee, and bring your left leg up to a ninety-degree angle. Use the strength of your left leg to stretch your right gluteal muscle. Hold and then repeat on the other side. You can also do this while standing and holding on to a piece of stable exercise equipment. Go into a squat and as you descend, cross one leg over the other knee, then use the squatting position to stretch the other leg's gluteal muscle. Squats are good for adding strength to your gluteal muscles. It's worth working with a trainer to make sure that you follow the right form for squats and other exercises.

One other important stretch for runners and bikers is for the hip flexors. Here your right knee is on the ground with your right leg flat on the ground and the sole of your right foot facing toward the ceiling. Your left leg is out in front of the right, bent at the knee with the foot flat on the ground. Your head and torso are straight up. Now you move your left knee forward until it comes to a ninety-degree angle just over your left foot. You will feel the stretch in your right groin area. One tweak is to raise your right arm straight up in the air to accentuate the stretch.

In addition, you must build the strength of your abdominal core and the muscles that run along your spinal column to stabilize your spinal vertebrae as you move. Traditional sit-ups—lying flat and straining to lift your body up by flexing upward and forward—are bad for your back. The "dead bug crawl" is a safer way to strengthen your abdominal muscles. While lying flat on your back, bend your knees up to your chest. Keep your abdominal muscles tight as you extend one leg out and bend the other leg up to your chest. Then switch and extend the other leg out. Try to keep your lower back flat against the floor and test this by having someone try to slip a hand under your back. Ideally, he or she won't be able to. Keep this bug crawl going for a while.

One-minute planks—resting on your forearms in a modified pushup position—are also effective. After thirty seconds you will begin to feel your abdominal muscles quiver as your core holds the pose. Try to hold this for a minute. You also can work your core with an exercise ball. There are many variations on plank exercises.

MUSCLE STRENGTHENING EXERCISES FOR RUNNERS AND BIKERS

Even when you take all the right precautions—whether you're a runner, a biker, or both—active athletes may still face some challenges. We need strong gluteal muscles, including the gluteus medius, and a strong core, to stabilize our hips, spine, and pelvis during running or biking. Many of us use compensatory motions to overcome weaknesses in these areas.

Think about how many strides we take during a run. If your cadence is 174 steps per minute and you run for forty-five minutes, that's 7,830 strides. That's plenty to inflame a sore Achilles tendon, or whatever ails you. Do you push off the ground with strong gluteals, like an Olympian, or are you using your quads to pull your legs forward? Do you know what it feels like to activate your gluteals? Can you feel them tighten on contraction or activation? If you lie on your side and raise your leg, and I try to push it down, how much resistance can you give? How strong are you?

Fortunately, many great exercises can strengthen your gluteus muscles and core. One is the single-leg squat with arms in runner pose (see Figure 6.5). This is an effective way to work the glutes in a running position. Stand tall on one leg, your "stance" leg, while bending your other leg and holding it off the floor. Lower into a squat with the stance leg. Repeat this ten times.

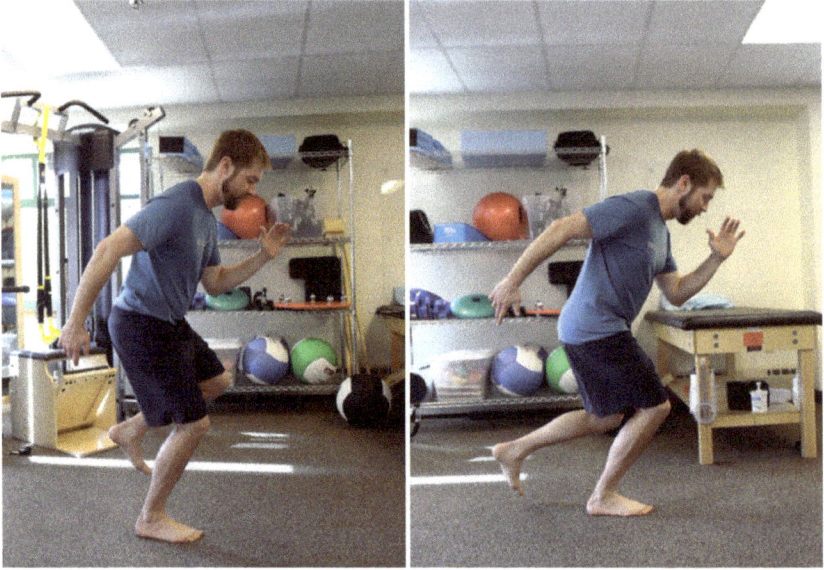

Figure 6.5: Single-leg squat.

There are a few things to watch for in your form as you tackle this exercise. Make sure the stance knee doesn't bend toward the raised leg, but rather goes straight up and down. The former indicates that your gluteal muscle on that side is weak. Secondly, watch that the knee of the stance leg does not extend too far forward as you bend this leg and squat. It may appear that the runner's knee is too far forward in the second photo of Figure 6.5, but if you notice the bend in his spine, you note that his back and lower leg are at the same angle or parallel. A friend can hold her hand in front of this knee to ensure that it doesn't flex forward too much and hit her hand.

Another way to practice this exercise is to stand with your buttocks about six inches away from a wall. Then start the exercise. As you sit into the squat using your glutes, your rear should just graze the wall.

The pelvic bridge (Figure 6.6) is another good gluteal muscle exercise and will give you a feel for the role of the gluteus muscle in stabilizing your pelvis. Lie on your back on a mat with your knees bent. Contract or squeeze your glutes to activate them as you raise your pelvis off the ground, as high as it goes. Now lift one leg in the air and extend it straight out in front of you, in line with your thigh and hip on that side.

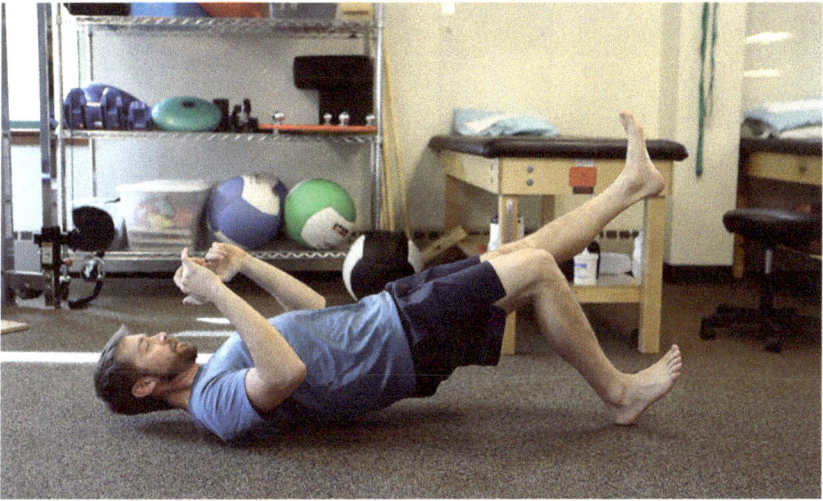

Figure 6.6: Single-leg pelvic bridge.

With the other leg, you work your gluteal muscle, the right one in these photos, as you lower your buttocks slowly to the ground. Pay careful attention as you do this. Is your pelvis level? Or does one leg drop lower than the other? You want to keep your pelvis level. You will feel some activation of your hamstrings, but try to keep them loose and focus on working your glutes. One tip for this is to keep the heel of the foot on the floor in contact with the floor with the toes raised, as shown in the photo, rather than the foot flat on the floor. This will help with gluteal rather than hamstring activation. Raise and lower on one side twelve times and then switch to the other side.

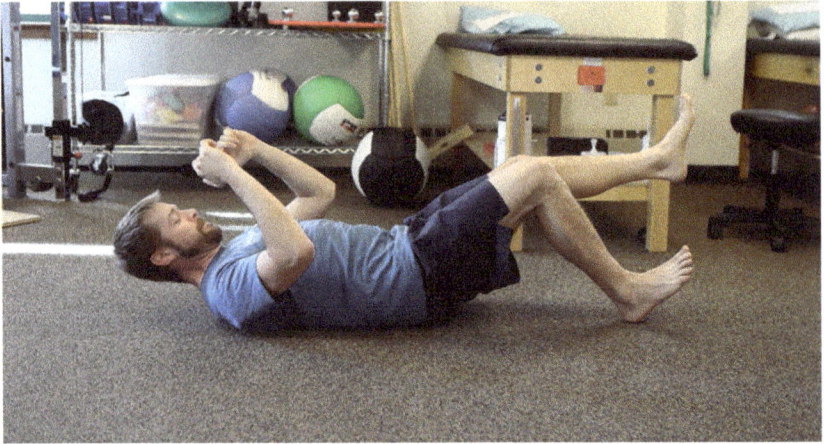

Figure 6.7: Completion of single-leg pelvic bridge exercise.

If this is too hard at first, you can activate your glutes and raise to a bridge using both legs (Figure 6.8). Once in the fully raised bridge with full gluteal activation (Figure 6.9) you would slowly lower both legs to the floor. When you have increased your strength such that you can do a few sets of these comfortably, then you can try the single-leg bridge.

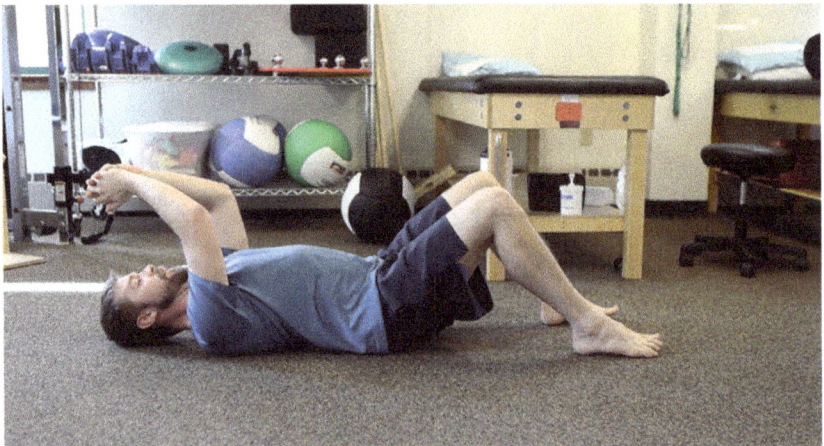

Figure 6.8: Beginning double-leg pelvic bridge.

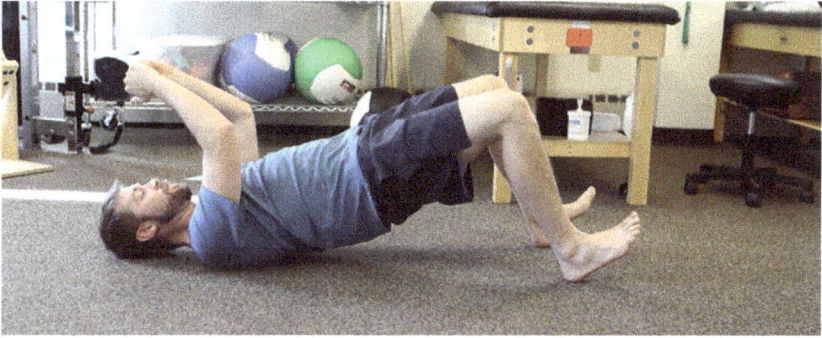

Figure 6.9: Double-leg pelvic bridge.

A smaller muscle that is very important is the gluteus medius. One of the most effective exercises for this is the clamshell. To challenge this muscle and build its strength we use a resistance band tied around your legs. You lie down and place the band around your thighs just above your knees. Then, you turn to your side with your knees bent and legs stacked together (Figure 7.0). You raise the top knee, keeping your feet together at the ankles (Figure 7.1), and lower it until you're in your original position with the legs touching again. We like to also engage your core by doing the exercise from a side plank position.

Most of us have weak core and gluteal muscles. We sit for much of our day

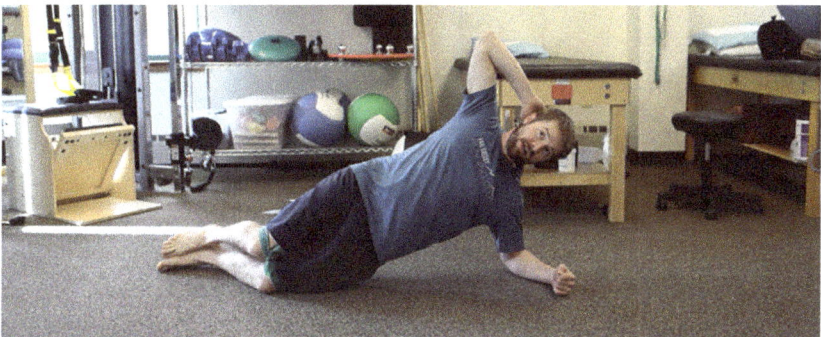

Figure 7.0: Clamshell exercise in side plank position.

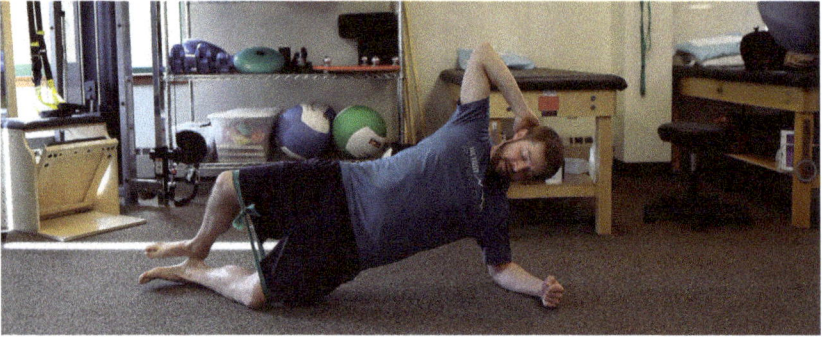

Figure 7.1: Spreading the legs in the clamshell

and we don't work these muscles. When we exercise, we overuse our quadriceps (thigh) muscles, a condition called "quad dominant." When we use our hip flexors instead of our gluteals we are cheating to get the work done. As an example, in the clamshell you want to work the gluteus medius. But often people engage their hip flexors instead. You should be able to press on the area of your hip flexor tendon and feel it soft and relaxed while you perform clamshells.

One way to overcome this is to contract your lower abdominals and engage them before raising your leg for the clamshell. To feel this, lie on your back. We are not looking to contract the middle and lower part of the rectus abdominus (the six pack in the middle), but the lower part between your navel and pubic bone. Try to engage and tighten this. It's a subtle movement.

Now try your clamshell with this lower abdominal engaged. You'll feel it more in your lateral buttocks muscle (gluteus medius) rather than your quads.

RUNNING GAIT ANALYSIS

I strongly recommend that those who have experienced challenges with their running gait undergo a running gait analysis. I talked about this in chapter 3. The examiner will give you a diagnosis and launch you on a gait therapy course.

Until someone experienced in gait analysis provides you specific insight, I can tell you a few don'ts. Don't try to do a self-correction at home. Don't read something or watch a video and try to change your gait. The most likely outcome of this is a nagging running injury. And injuries mean a setback to regular exercise.

You might watch a YouTube video of a skilled younger runner telling you to land on your midfoot with a cadence of 180 steps per minute. If you are a heel striker with a cadence of 172, that's fine. Don't try to change this, certainly not all at once. Again, we are more interested in where your foot lands in relation to your body. There have been and will be many excellent competitive heel-striking runners.

If you want to play with gait changes, go to a track and try a small distance trial like four hundred meters (one lap on a track) or eight hundred meters. But don't try something different for your entire six-mile run. You're asking for it.

Don't watch online videos about kicking up your heels as a warm-up exercise or part of your run. If your motion is correct, your leg will follow after the glutes push off. If you just activate your hamstrings to kick up your heels toward your buttocks, to simulate good runners, you might end up with a hamstring pull.

• • •

Cycling comes with its own joys and challenges. It's a passion for me. It's particularly alluring in the mountains of Colorado. As we mentioned in chapter 3, those of you who do more biking than running should do a lactate threshold test on a special stationary bike.

Your graphs will be similar to the examples above. And the training plan will be similar but tailored more toward cycling. But in general, the goals for cyclists are the same as those for runners: shifting the curve and building larger and more plentiful mitochondria.

Fortunately, in biking it is not as easy to injure ourselves with our form. We are not impacting the ground with our body, and this lessens injuries compared to running. That doesn't, of course, eliminate other potential accidents or problems.

We can still exhibit poor form on a bike, such as favoring a stronger leg, just like in running. If you have done spin classes you have likely done an exercise where you take one foot off the pedal and use only one foot, then switch sides. This can clue you in to imbalances.

Some of our patients complain of back pain with biking. If you have muscle tension in your lower back, there are two areas to evaluate. One is the fit of the bike—the seat height, handlebar height, frame size, etc. The other is if you are straining too much to do the work. For example, if your gluteals are not strong enough for the hill you are climbing, or the resistance you apply on your spinning bike, you will engage your hip flexors to get the work done. Some of the hip flexors are connected to the lower lumbar spine, and you will feel lower back tension with the workout.

If you engage your core and your gluteals as you pedal up a steep hill, you will feel the gluteals working, and how it differs from your typical form. During a ride, bring your arms higher on the handlebar to allow you to sit more upright. Then extend your spine backward. This should relax your lower spine. If it's too sore and hard to relax and extend, you are working too hard based on your current conditioning. You'll get there—but give it some time to build your strength.

Spinning classes are a good cardio workout, especially in bad weather, but they do not replace miles on an outdoor bike. Indoor cycles are mounted on a frame, firmly grounded to the floor. As such they do not require the balance, and therefore, the core work involved in cycling outdoors.

• • •

Regardless of precautions, we all sometimes get injured. It can be difficult to face up to this. One of the interesting aspects of an injury is determining the underlying cause. For example, right hip pain may come from compensating for a problem that is actually on the left side.

What happens to our fitness if, due to injury, we can't engage in our sport of choice? This is where cross-training comes in. Depending on your injury, biking may be a good alternative, along with indoor variations such as spinning classes, stationary bikes, or at-home options such as a Peloton bike with a web-based app that lets you remotely participate in a spin class. Even if an injury doesn't sideline you, too-frequent workouts such as running might cause excessive inflammation. Being able to mix in some good bike rides will keep you fit.

Finally, if something ails you, don't hesitate to see a physical therapist. I suffered an entire summer with Achilles tendinitis. This led to a loss of balance in my gait and subsequent hip pain that sidelined me on a run. I had to walk home for the first time in my life.

Once I got into physical therapy, I asked myself why I hadn't had the sense to stop sooner and get help.

For those who are not yet 2.0 athletes, and have not embraced regular workouts as described here, you will need to get accustomed to heavy breathing and fatigue. Many trainers have their own way of expressing this, but the idea is that to advance in aerobic training you have to push yourself to a point where it is uncomfortable to breathe. Much of your work will be just below this level of exertion, where you can speak, but in running intervals and on race day you need to accept the discomfort and push yourself. Think back to childhood when, and if, you learned how to swim. At one point you probably practiced swimming underwater. Do you remember what it felt like when you finally gave up and surfaced for air? That's the uncomfortable breathing that I'm talking about. Similarly, endurance running is about pushing your own envelope, adding miles gradually to your long run as you train for distance.

To weekend warriors or even some seasoned athletes, the various techniques and approaches I advise here may seem like a lot of bother. Some of them may not apply to you at all. But I am certain that if you follow through with the lactate threshold testing and other approaches that suit you, you will morph into a better, fitter version of yourself. You will be at the 2.0 level. And some of you may be poised to proceed to the exalted 3.0 level.

CHAPTER SEVEN

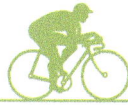

SUPPLEMENTS: WHAT DO YOU REALLY NEED?

What role should nutritional supplements play in our diets? Similar to the old Beatles song, "all you need is love," we could add, "and a healthy diet." In most situations, as we will discuss, a plant-based diet will provide what your body needs for optimal health. But I will discuss some helpful supplements for your overall well-being, as well as improved athletic performance, in this chapter.

One major challenge in a discussion of supplements is that they are not regulated by the Food and Drug Administration the way prescription medications are. No clinical trials are required to prove their effectiveness. Many people have opinions about the benefits of supplements—opinions that are not based on science. Even in the world of evidence-based medicine, where we look for clinical trials to guide us, there is a lot of confusion in the studies. Some of them lack scientific rigor.

For example, many of us familiar with different studies on Vitamin E supplementation understand the challenges of conflicting conclusions. One year it appears to be a good idea to take vitamin E and another year, it's not. A daily aspirin is thought to reduce the risk of heart attack and stroke, yet some studies suggest the negatives outweigh the positives.

Physicians interested in nutrition like to think of food as a medicine. We've discussed how switching to a plant-based diet can relieve chest pain or angina in patients with heart disease in as little as two weeks. The foods we encourage you to eat as part of the Vail Method all play a role in healing the body. A plant-based diet reduces the risk of heart disease and other chronic degenerative disorders.

Before addressing any concern about what supplements to take, I encourage you to return to the basics of what you need to eat as reviewed in chapters 4 and 5. Adequate consumption of macronutrients—carbohydrates, protein, and fats—is important. How many calories do you need for your level of activity? How many grams of carbohydrates and protein? The timing of consumption of carbs and proteins should never be underestimated, particularly for those of us getting primed for running or other sports. You have to replenish your glycogen storage before exercise, for example, and during prolonged exercise longer than forty-five minutes or an hour.

IMPROVED ATHLETIC PERFORMANCE: ERGOGENIC SUPPLEMENTS

As we weigh the possible value of supplements from a sports nutrition perspective, we are especially interested in *ergogenic* products. An ergogenic supplement refers to one that helps prepare you for exercise, improves your exercise performance, and/or aids in recovery from exercise. Again, I would emphasize that the main way to get ready for exercise is getting adequate calories, carbohydrates, and protein. Carbohydrates are a proven ergogenic aid. Water is the most critical ergogenic aid. Since adequate hydration is so important, water needs to be replaced during exercise. These are the keys to great athletic performance and good health.

Some athletes nonetheless find supplements to be helpful ergogenics. Caffeine is a good example. A stimulant, it has been proven to have ergogenic properties. It increases energy expenditure, speed, and power in cyclists, and boosts repeated sprint performances in runners.[39] Gels are also popular among some long-distance runners and bikers. If you read the labels of gels sold for consumption during prolonged exercise, you will see that most of them are carbohydrates or sugars combined with caffeine.

There are also athletes who rely on supplements to buttress their protein intake. Again, as I pointed out in chapter 4, recreational athletes should not need a protein supplement. Elite competitive athletes, on the other hand, may struggle to consume sufficient calories and nutrients from food alone.

One of the building blocks of protein that is important to replace after exercise is *leucine*, one of the three branched-chain amino acids (BCAAs). We need approximately three grams, or three thousand milligrams. If you are using a post exercise protein supplement such as a pea and rice blend or whey, check the label. It should contain adequate leucine and other BCAAs.

Creatine monohydrate is one of the most tested and proven ergogenic nutritional supplements. It increases exercise capacity and muscle mass and has been proven safe. To start using creatine and build the level in the body, 0.3 grams per kilogram per day are taken for five to seven days. That should be followed by a maintenance dose of 5 to 7 grams per day.[40]

Many supplements promise to raise your *testosterone* level. None is as effective as taking testosterone itself. While not a nutritional supplement, it is an important hormone to maintain at physiologic levels. Testosterone impacts general health and sports performance. It helps build muscle and increase energy. We can think of it as a hormonal supplement. We encourage Vail Method participants to have their testosterone levels tested as part of a general health checkup. As we discussed in chapter 3, when levels are low, testosterone replacement is a proven and successful strategy. It is preferable to replace testosterone to physiologic levels than to supplement with hormone precursors such as DHEA.

Beta-hydroxy-beta-methylbutyrate (HMB) is another supplement some athletes favor. A metabolite, or breakdown product of leucine, it is proven to increase muscle mass by 0.5–1.0 kilograms over three to six weeks.[41] The dosage for HMB is 1.5–3.0 kilograms per day. But you should be aware that there is considerable debate whether athletes should use HMB. Good diets—such as the type of plant-based regime we advocate in the Vail Method—include adequate protein and thus should preclude the consumption of HMB.[42]

Ginseng is an herbal supplement sold in numerous varieties: Asian, Korean, Chinese, American, and Canadian. It has been studied extensively as something that potentially increases athletic endurance. Research has shown that it raises aerobic capacity by decreasing lactate production, thus increasing running time. One scientific review[43] summarizes ten studies on ginseng. The majority of the studies show these benefits.

Turmeric, a spice that a lot of athletes and nutritionists like to consume, has become all the rage. A key ingredient in curries, it is sold in root form, similar to ginger, and can be shaved and added to salads and other foods. Turmeric contains curcumin, which may have beneficial anti-inflammatory properties that can reduce muscle soreness after exercise. Thus, it could be considered ergogenic in terms of enhancing recovery.

SUPPLEMENTS WITH GENERAL HEALTH BENEFITS

I have been focusing on the use of supplements for sports perfor-mance, but want you to be aware of their other beneficial effects. Turmeric is a good example. Besides the anti-inflammatory proper-ties for sports recovery that I cited above, it is believed to be helpful for patients with irritable bowel disease, among other ailments.[44]

For women dealing with side effects of menopause, certain herbs act as *phytoestrogens* and can relieve these symptoms. Examples include dong quai, chasteberry, black cohosh, ginseng, and licorice root.[45] Soy is also a phytoestrogen. The heavy consumption of soy in Asia helps explain the reduced complaints of menopausal symptoms among women in that part of the world.

In terms of vitamins, *B12* is an essential supplement for people following a plant-based diet. B12 or cyanocobalamin is mostly obtained from meat and is difficult to obtain from foods eaten on a vegan diet. However, some plant foods, such as nori, do contain B12, which may explain why many Japanese people eat small pieces of nori for breakfast.[46] I take a 2,500-microgram B12 lozenge once a week.

Also, depending on your sun exposure, *Vitamin D3* supplements may be beneficial. Your blood level of Vitamin D can be tested easily at the time of your yearly checkup. I have used Vitamin D capsules, but only sporadically. I get plenty of sun where I live in Colorado. With three hundred days of sunlight a year, Colorado is sometimes referred to as the other sunshine state.

Omega-3 fatty acids are important to include in your diet as well. They play a positive role in brain health. In my own diet, flaxseeds, shelled hemp seeds, and chia seeds are the primary sources of omega-3 fatty acids. These are all short chain but converted by the body into long chain fatty acids. I grind the flaxseeds in my blender and sprinkle them into my oatmeal or sprouted grain cereal. I sprinkle a table-spoon of hemp hearts and chia seeds into my super salad at lunch. I also add a quarter-cup of walnuts—another source of omega-3 fatty acids—to my morning steel-cut oatmeal. I supplement it with Algae Omega by Nordic Natural. It is a vegetarian source providing 715 milligrams of omega-3s per serving.

To lower "bad" LDL cholesterol, following the kind of plant-based diet we advocate in the Vail Method works well. Oats, barley, whole grains, and beans are high in soluble fiber that binds and lowers cholesterol. The same is true for fruits such as apples, strawberries, and citrus, which contain soluble fiber known as pectin that provides the same benefit.

Some supplements used for lowering "bad" LDL cholesterol are *plant sterols* and *stanols*. They are naturally occurring compounds found in the same foods described above. A two-gram supplement of plant sterols can lower LDL cholesterol 6 to 12 percent.[47] I used this successfully (Meta-Sitosterol 2.0 by Metagenics) while I was transitioning to a plant-based diet. Once I made the transition, my total cholesterol dropped to 150 and my LDL to 86. With those numbers, I no longer needed the supplement.

It can be a challenge to weigh the advantages versus the disadvantages of a treatment with statin drugs, particularly in borderline situations such as moderately elevated cholesterol. In chapter 3, I offered some tests we use to help make that choice.

The Vail Method focuses more on a healthy lifestyle, exercise, and a plant-based diet to help reduce inflammation in your body, as well as the risk of heart attack, stroke, and cancer. This is a more effective strategy than trying to take antioxidant supplements to reduce inflammation or help ward off disease caused by poor diet and lifestyle choices. This is much the same as patients we work with who want a magical pair of running shoes to fix their ailments or pains, when what they really need is to work on their physical therapy exercises.

My own thinking and life experiences have led me to the conclusion that a whole-food plant-based diet will provide most of the vitamins and minerals that the majority of people need for good health. Look at the abundance of calcium in vegetables. Nature has everything that we need—if we just look for it.

CHAPTER EIGHT

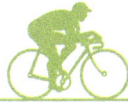

MINDFULNESS: TELLING YOUR MIND TO SHUT THE F*** UP

M ake time to still your mind on a regular basis! It's one of the essentials for a healthy lifestyle. I've already hit you over the head with the importance of a good plant-based diet and consistent exercise regimen as cornerstones of getting fit and staying healthy as you enter middle age and beyond. In the Vail Method, mindfulness plays a crucial role too.

It makes sense if you stop and think about it. Most of our day-to-day lives can be compared to an eight-legged arthropod. The various tentacles are constantly tugging in different directions. Work. Family life. Chores. Commuting. Just dealing with life and all of its challenges. They all consume enormous amounts of time, energy, and emotion. Now we're asking you to sign on to the Vail Method and potentially devote even more time and energy to diet and exercise.

And, all the while, your mind is racing. The worries quickly pile up. They may be related to your business. Or any of a hundred issues that occupy your thoughts—issues at work, at home, with finances, children, or older parents. There are so many concerns to occupy our thoughts and distract us from living in the moment.

When the mind churns like that, it affects your body and health. Many people turn to the equivalent of a glass of wine, a drink, or in Colorado and other states, marijuana, to try to relieve that stress.

In medicine, we understand the placebo response. This occurs when patients are given a placebo but told it is a medicine that will help them, and they feel relief from their problems. This is a perfect illustration of the mind-body connection, an important concept for you to understand for your health, particularly as you figure out the best ways to calm your mind. As the placebo example illustrates, the human mind can help with healing. But it also can cause harm to our physical health. Stomach ulcers and gastric reflux are good examples, but many other diseases are worsened by stress and anxiety. We often see this connection in irritable bowel syndrome, where nothing can be found physically wrong with the intestines, yet someone can be terribly sick.

And, of course, these stresses and anxieties affect our sleep. If your mind is racing with questions or issues when you go to bed, or when you wake up in the middle of the night, you're going to have a hard time falling to sleep or returning back to sleep. This begins a vicious cycle. You won't be well rested. How can you perform well at work or at endurance exercise if you're exhausted?

I know this from my own experience. I have a busy medical practice that keeps me at work for ten-hour days on a regular basis.

Devoting time to my family is important to me. And so is keeping up a very active exercise regime—long runs and bike rides three to four days a week. I also prepare many of my plant-based meals. It takes a lot of discipline to keep this all moving forward daily.

Schedules like this are the stuff of stress. And stress is a major killer. It doesn't get mentioned with heart disease or cancer, but it plays a role in all that ails us. It permeates our jobs and lives so profoundly that we don't recognize it. How many of our country's presidents had dark hair at the start of their terms and ended up much grayer or white-haired by the end?

Biofeedback is another illustration of the mind-body connection. It has been used to help patients with disorders in which stress and other conditions play a key role—such as migraine headaches, chronic pain, and high blood pressure. A doctor or technician uses different sensors to measure your heart rate, brain waves, skin temperature, sweating, or muscle contraction. The sensors used depend on the condition you're experiencing. For example, brain waves are measured with an EEG or electroencephalogram.

Software then allows the examiner to make you aware of these physiological functions. This might be as simple showing you the change in your heart rate when you are experiencing a particular condition. It could also be more complex—such as training patients with attention deficit hyperactivity disorder to change the pattern of their brain waves. It helps you be in touch with the intricate ways in which the mind and the body are intimately connected. You become aware of your physiological state and reaction to stress. With that kind of knowledge, you can take control of relaxing your mind without the need for technology.

So, how do we control the stresses that affect us? How do we address the anxieties not as a placebo would, but in a substantive, helpful way? Mindfulness, or mental relaxation, is the best way I know. Just like taking a day off from exercise after a big race or heavy workout, resting the mind allows you to appreciate what you have been doing and regroup. From my work with the Vail Method, I see a common denominator behind meditation, relaxation, and calming the body during heavy aerobic exercise, and in moments of career performance stress. That common factor is proper breathing—being aware of your breath and how to calm it.

As we increase exercise output and effort, our breathing becomes labored. Coaches will often speak of calming our bodies by focusing on our breath. Sometimes in running we specify a certain number of breaths per number of footsteps.

Similarly, in surgery, I sometimes catch myself taking a slower, cleansing breath right before a critical maneuver, much as a sharp-shooter does before pulling the trigger.

Many approaches to mindfulness also focus on breathing. Mindfulness has become popular in the US in the past few years. It seems that almost everybody is exploring different paths to it. For some people, meditation works well. Many also use yoga as a way to calm their minds and stretch their muscles at the same time.

For still others, communing with nature does the trick. That can be as easy as a simple walk in the park with or without a dog. It can be fly fishing, horseback riding, skiing, or any number of other outdoor activities. In the mountains of Colorado, where I live, nature is so bountiful and ubiquitous that exploring it to find your inner self is almost a way of life. The spectacular trails, the gushing rivers and streams, the Rockies rising up around us: it all makes for an incredible backdrop for a foray into mindfulness.

If you're cerebral, you may find the solace of mindfulness in written or spoken journals. This may also be a helpful tip to relieve your mind of thinking about something you need to do, so that you don't rehash it before sleep. In my experience, there is no right way to calm the mind. The important thing is that it relaxes and distracts you. As you explore the various avenues to mindfulness, you will find that breath control is a thread that runs through many if not all of them.

Meditation has worked well for me, and research supports its health benefits. I've experimented and found that the easiest way to begin is by sitting in a relaxed position, closing my eyes, taking slow, long, deep, deliberate breaths, and exhaling similarly. I pay close attention to my breathing. And I learned I don't have to sit cross-legged on the floor. Sitting in a chair may be more comfortable for longer periods.

Try to go for two minutes with a quiet mind, then try to build to five minutes, then at least ten minutes. It's a great way to end your morning stretching session, and well worth getting up just a little bit earlier to do.

If you're an outdoors type, you may prefer a spot in nature for meditation. Find a comfortable place in your backyard, or on your porch or deck, close your eyes, and see how it feels. Parks and quiet spaces—ubiquitous even in urban neighborhoods—can also make good meditation places.

Some meditators prefer guidance from a professional who is versed in meditation techniques to help usher them through the process. Particularly if you are new to the whole concept, a guided approach is a good way to get you engaged in it. Thanks to the boom in the mindfulness movement in the US, there are a lot of meditation centers and teachers to choose from. Especially if you live in a city, you won't have to look far for a center offering regular sessions.

There are also several excellent guided meditation apps available for your smartphone or computer. Here are three of the top options:

Deepak Chopra (www.deepakchopra.com): One of the best-known public figures in the New Age movement, Chopra has helped popularize meditation in American culture. He has teamed with Oprah Winfrey to produce a series of guided twenty-one-day sessions. More recently he has produced these by himself. The sessions are offered online several times a year. All you have to do is register and sign in daily and block out a small slice of your day. CD sets of the sessions are also available.

The themes of the sessions vary widely and include subjects like Expanding Your Happiness, Creating Abundance, Energy of Attraction, and Youthful Energy. Over the course of the three weeks, Winfrey and Deepak examine the general theme from a different perspective every day. Then they guide you through the daily meditation.

Each daily session typically starts with Winfrey giving a two- to three-minute pep talk on the day's topic. Chopra then explores the topic in greater depth and gives a meditating mantra for the day. Finally, he walks you through the basics of meditation, explains proper posture and breathing, and offers tips to keep your mind from wandering. The meditation follows, accompanied by soothing background music. Each session lasts around fifteen minutes.

In my experience, Chopra's meditations are almost always thoughtful. They offer a way to calm your mind and start the day. They also offer a great perspective on life and happiness. For example, he recently defined our sense of fulfilment as when our lives have meaning: love, purpose, achievement, self-esteem, positive core beliefs, and trust in a higher power.

Headspace (www.headspace.com): This is another highly popular app, available on your smartphone or any device. It is hosted by Andy Puddicombe, a former Buddhist monk turned meditation teacher.

Like Chopra, Puddicombe starts each daily session with a primer in meditation. His biggest focus is also on breathing. He then guides you through a meditation session lasting around ten minutes.

The first ten sessions are free. The sessions available vary from quick one-minute meditations to more in-depth sessions of up to twenty minutes. Aside from the general meditation, there are special categories that focus on certain themes, such as stress, anxiety, or change. One category that may be of particular interest to Vail Method devotees focuses directly on meditation as it relates to sports. It includes subcategories for those who want to key in on topics such as motivation, training, and recovery.

As an app, Headspace.com is well designed and easy to use. It works best for beginners to meditation. It's also great for those on the run who want to fit a daily mindfulness session into their schedules.

Insight Timer (www.Insighttimer.com): This app features more than eleven thousand meditations. They cover a wide range of themes, from "Nidra Yoga for Sleep" to "Morning Gratitude." While the Deepak Chopra and Headspace options are guided by the same voices, Insight Timer features a diverse range of guides and voices.

The approach is similar to the other two apps. In most cases, the guide starts by talking you through the basics of mediation, concentrating on the techniques of breathing and focusing the mind. Already comfortable with the basics? Many of the sessions are at intermediate and advanced levels.

For those who want to explore meditation in greater depth, Insight Timer offers access to dozens of lectures and courses. It's a good opportunity to explore how the various approaches to meditation differ from each other. An eager student can choose a meditation teacher from some of the best-known names in the field. Most everything offered on Insight Timer is complimentary.

• • •

More and more Americans are also practicing yoga as a path to mindfulness. Novices should be aware that there are more than a dozen types of it. The distinctions can be important. Four of the most popular include:

1. *Hatha* is by far the best known. It's considered introductory level. Many yoga centers offer starter courses in Hatha.

2. *Vinyasa* is more intense physically.

3. *Ashtanga,* the so-called eight-limb approach, is for the more advanced yogi.

4. *Kundalini* is known for its emphasis on blending mediation, including chants and mantras, together with stretching.

Yoga enthusiasts consider it much more than another type of exercise. For many of them, it's also an effective form of mind-body intervention, something to help cope with stress and depression. Many studies have shown yoga's effectiveness in alleviating depression. In some of them, yoga has demonstrated an ability to relieve hypercortisolemia —the heightened levels of stress frequently seen in depression—and reduce other parameters of stress.[48]

Like meditation, yoga is easily accessible and widely available.

Even before we start experimenting with which approach to mindfulness works best, there are a couple of easy practices all of us can adopt to help calm our minds. One big way to help enter a state of mindfulness—and eventually get better sleep—is to avoid checking emails at night. In our wired world, stimulation from electronic devices tends to disturb our peace of mind and sleep. Shutting off your devices early in the evening will go a long way in helping you have a restful night. If you regularly take a laptop into your bed, break the habit.

Another thing we can do is learn is how to be more grateful and appreciative. I know, that sounds like a basic commandment. But as a doctor, I have observed that a lot of anxiety stems from a lack of appreciation for what we have. This is seen in a number of depression and anxiety patients. One helpful concept taught in leadership courses is to start your day with five imaginary coins in your pocket. During the day you acknowledge people for their work and good deeds, removing one of the imaginary coins each time. By the end of the day, your pocket should be empty.

At Thanksgiving, many families go around the table and ask each person to describe what they are thankful for. It's often funny and sad at the same time to watch teenagers struggle to come up with something meaningful, or simply repeat something someone else says. Unfortunately, adults can be the same way.

You can start with being grateful for each day. Be thankful for the people who care about you. Be grateful if you are fortunate to have someone who "gets you" and then tolerates you. When you have inner peace and happiness, this will come naturally to you.

Above all, we should all learn to live in the moment, not putting things off for the future, dreaming about it, or regretting the past. For almost three decades, I have cared for senior citizens as an ophthalmologist and learned that we don't know when our time is up. Clearly genetics plays an important role in our lives and longevity. Many contemporary researchers believe we can beat our genetics and live longer, stronger lives. There is some truth to this.

Quality of life is important, not just quantity. We see seniors who smoke cigarettes like fiends, eat fatty, greasy food and animal meats, and live long lives. Over the years I have questioned these patients and often there is no answer or logical explanation for their longevity. But I have seen a difference in the quality of their health and their energy level, compared to those living an active, healthy lifestyle as we teach in the Vail Method. There is much more to what I wish for you in my program—it's not just about living longer than average; it's about living it energetically and enjoying a fulfilled life too.

No one can predict the winning lottery numbers or the future. This is why it's important to stop dreaming of a better day and instead be as satisfied and content as you can in the present. Similarly, it is only self-punishment to live regretting the past and things you wished you had done. We must all learn to live in the moment.

Not long ago a sixty-year-old man came to the University of Colorado Boulder's Human Performance Lab with a goal: optimizing his marathon time. In his next race, he made an impressive improvement in time. Sadly, a few weeks after the race, he was hit by a car and died.

The moral for me? What is more essential than meditation or any other mindfulness technique is learning to live in the present and enjoy your life.

CHAPTER NINE

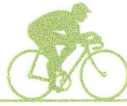

REST, SLEEP, AND RECOVERY: GIVING YOUR BODY THE DOWNTIME IT REQUIRES

fter pushing you to step up your running, biking, and all-around athletic game, I'm giving you a new assignment: see how long you can lounge on the couch. Just kidding. Or half kidding. The truth in that jest is that any successful exercise regime must incorporate regular periods of rest and recuperation.

As you are aware by now, for the Vail Method, consistent, hard training is nonnegotiable. That training will not produce the results you want, however, unless it's coupled with adequate periods of rest. As we have hammered home throughout the book, the method is designed to nudge your aerobic workout capacity to higher limits over an extended period. The plan is designed to constantly guide you to the next performance level, whether you are running, biking, or doing other forms of exercise. If you're running for forty-five minutes, we want you to extend to one-hour sessions. In your interval work and on race day, we are looking for improved results times for you, based on your goals.

The goal of training like this is to induce a stress. At its best it will be a stress that allows you to build stronger muscles. If you go too far, your progress and performance could go in the wrong direction. To keep that from happening, you will have to learn when to reel it in to let your muscles recover.

Football and soccer players are well versed in this kind of work hard and rest hard schedule. They train intensely during the season. Then, in the off-season, they take a break from the rigors of intense workouts. In the extended off periods, they typically follow a lower-key workout regime or engage in other sports. In many cases, their off-season downtime can continue for three months or more. This break is programmed so they can rebound and be more prepared when the season starts. Those of you who regularly compete in marathons or other running or cycling races probably follow a version of this approach as well. It's not uncommon for marathoners to ratchet up the heavy training in the weeks leading up to a race. Then they ease back just before and afterwards.

But giving your body the rest it needs means more than taking pre- and post-race timeouts. You will need to schedule in downtime between heavy workouts, build in light days, take workout holidays, and more. Most important, you must become aware of when you are overtraining, overworking, or just not getting enough shut-eye or mental repose. Your body usually talks to you. When something is slightly off it might communicate with a whisper. But if the body is way overworked, you can expect something more akin to a scream.

Learn to be aware of the signals the body sends. Are you feeling too tired but pushing yourself to move forward with a workout? Been there. Often, after I perform a surgery, I'll try to get a ride in up the mountain to unwind and maintain my workout schedule. When you're feeling a need for a cup of coffee before you start exercise, that's a hint. You can also learn to read your body. What do your legs feel like? What percentage of your strength and energy is there? Are you off your game? Really off?

Apart from exercising too heavily, many recreational athletes overextend themselves in all aspects of their lives, including work and home life. In particular, working professionals often try to get by on five hours of sleep a night. They wake too early. They then work ten hours a day—fifty hours a week or more. And after work, when they know they are tired, they try to force a training run or gym workout.

Even those who get sufficient rest sometimes do too much high-intensity training. And on top of that, due to poor nutritional advice, they restrict their carb intake way too much, failing to understand that carbs are needed for good workouts. No wonder they are not getting the results they want.

Recreational athletes should take a page from their elite athlete counterparts. Elite athletes—those who perform professionally or semiprofessionally—tend to value their sleep. They train when they are rested. Their training is often focused on longer, moderately paced distances—the midzone category of aerobics that I discussed in chapter 6. On days that they feel off or too tired, they switch away from hard-driven aerobics to a core workout or gym exercise.

I'll give you a recent example of how I had to get in tune with the messages my own body was sending. Not long ago, I traveled to London and Paris for eight days. I did some running during the trip, but nothing like the schedule I like to keep when I am at home. When I returned, I was jet-lagged. For the first two days I couldn't have considered running, I was too tired. But on the third morning I went out for a run. I thought I did well. My pace was good. I came home and got ready for work, and when I walked out to my car it felt like someone had pulled the plug out of me. The normal bounce in my step was gone.

Two days later I tried again. This time I noticed my heart rate was below normal even though I was moving well at the beginning. But by 2.5 miles my battery was running low. I stopped to walk a bit, which I almost never do. I started up again, but stopped again shortly after. By 3.5 miles I hung it up and returned to my car.

I was convinced that my heart rate monitor must have a weak or dying battery. Even when I was moving at my normal pace, my heart rate lagged. These are signs to watch for in your own aerobics. One day later I biked up a steep mountain road with a friend and felt fine. By Sunday, I had a decent run. Two days after that, all was back to normal—heart rate, pace, and so on. That cycle of getting back on schedule following my trip took all of nine days.

I think it would be helpful to look more closely at the reasons why overtraining or general work fatigue impact us so heavily. Several of my colleagues in physiology have done great research in this area.

With fatigue and overtraining, your lactate threshold levels (which we discussed in chapter 6) begin to fall. The lactate curve shifts to the left. Your muscle glycogen storage starts to decline. This is a major problem. When your muscle glycogen gets depleted you have more protein utilization and muscle catabolism—muscle damage that might interfere with your glycogen storage. As your muscle glycogen gets depleted, your muscle cells release less calcium, which reduces the force output of the muscle. In the end, it decreases your endurance, sometimes dramatically.

As you may recall from earlier chapters, we can measure the

glycogen in your muscles with a simple ultrasound test. The glycogen levels measured have been correlated to muscle biopsies by Inigo San Millan, PhD, the Colorado-based physiologist who has done excellent research in this area.

In some cases, decreased muscle glycogen turns out to be more a function of inadequate food intake than fatigue. These are exceptions, instances we can address with nutrition counseling. But for the vast majority of others, the drop in glycogen results from too much exercise, too many hard workouts with insufficient rest in between. In short, they happen when you push the body too hard.

Monitoring muscle glycogen is an excellent way to assess nutrition and overtraining. Sometimes after races we see drops so significant, they can take several days or longer to recover. Elite athletes who compete in different time zones will see decreases in muscle glycogen from distant travel.

For athletes who have serious overtraining issues, one result is decreased hemoglobin levels. Within all humans, red blood cells continually die and drop out of circulation while new red blood cells are reproduced. Athletes who over-train do not produce enough red blood cells. Consequently, their hemoglobin drops. And since it is hemoglobin that carries oxygen, the result is a decreased oxygen supply. Just a one-point drop in hemoglobin equates to a 5 to 7 percent decrease in blood oxygen carrying capacity. The result: the athlete loses his snap.

In contrast, hemoglobin can work to the advantage of athletes who train in high-altitude areas. The reason: hemoglobin and hematocrit rise at high altitudes. That, in turn, increases the blood-carrying capacity of oxygen. This explains why athletes who train in high-altitude areas and compete at sea level perform so well. Many of the top finishers in the Boston, New York, and other marathons train in the mountains of Ethiopia, Peru, or the Himalayas.

So, what are the best ways to help the body recover? While sitting on the couch might be tempting, it's not the ideal way to spend your downtime.

Some professional and recreational athletes use the periodization approach to bring balance to their workouts. This refers to strategic implementation of specific training phases. Typically, in periodization, training is broken down into micro workouts with varying levels of intensity. There are different schools of periodization but one that makes most sense to me is divided into four categories: endurance, intensity, competition, and recovery. The length of time for each varies, depending on the individual and his or her goals. The built-in recovery phase takes the guesswork out of when or even how long you should allow yourself to recover after heavy training or a race. Following competition and recovery, you can restart the cycle. Studies have shown that this approach has a positive effect on muscle strength.

We encourage Vail Method participants to approach the sports recovery period in the same smart, artful way that we approach every other aspect of the program. Above all, don't be sedentary or get in a cycle where you put on pounds. Use downtime as an opportunity to engage in an activity that is different from your main sport. Runners should use the opening to pursue cycling, for example, and vice versa. Swimmers can take a break and delve into yoga. It's a moment to try something you have thought about but did not have the time to try. Pilates may have captured your interest. Now's the time to pursue it.

At the very least, use the downtime to engage more intensely in the kind of deep stretching and muscle-building exercises that your day-to-day schedule doesn't accommodate.

In the end, the two important things to remember about

downtime are: respect it and incorporate it into your workout regimes, and be creative about finding fun and useful ways to best spend your downtime.

THE CRITICAL REJUVENATION OF SLEEP

Along with adhering to a solid diet, exercising regularly, and paying attention to mindfulness, getting a good night's sleep is one of the most important tenets of maintaining good health. This is something you've heard over and over but it bears repeating here. That's why I made getting sound sleep a pillar of the Vail Method. I cannot emphasize enough the negative effects of sleep deprivation and the benefits of sleeping soundly on a nightly basis. On a personal level, I have found that a healthy approach to sleep is the basis for all other pursuits. It's crucial to my ability to maintain a busy medical practice, keep up an active running and biking regime, and be an attentive father and husband.

As I doctor, I have witnessed firsthand the negative side effects of sleep deprivation in my patients. Poor sleep, according to a number of studies, aggravates all kinds of health problems, including heart disease and other chronic diseases, weakens the immune system, disturbs blood sugar metabolism, and increases inflammation and depression. Of course, I am not saying that sleep is a cure-all. But, clearly, it's part of the foundation for preventing these and other health woes.

Maintaining good sleeping habits, in contrast, has been shown to have a remarkably positive impact on many aspects of health, both short term and long term. Sleep is good for your general memory and perceptiveness. It's also great for your heart health, metabolism, and immune system. Those who follow the Vail Method, with its emphasis on regular exercise, will find that sound sleep every night maximizes athletic performance, including speed, accuracy, and reaction times.

The Vail Method health assessment includes questions relating to sleep. We want to know the basics of your sleeping habits: How many hours of sleep do you get? How many times do you wake up? Are you rested or exhausted when you awake? Do you snore? Has your bed partner observed you sitting up, or gasping for air? Has he or she observed you go from loud snoring to a pause in breathing?

A "yes" to the last few questions suggests possible sleep apnea, which can be life-threatening. Traditionally sleep apnea is diagnosed by having the patient spend a night at a sleep lab as described in chapter 3.

Fortunately, some excellent sleep apnea treatment options are available, including simple weight loss, a change in sleeping position, an oral appliance, and use of a continuous positive airway pressure (CPAP) machine.

The last two options may not be familiar to you. An oral appliance is similar to a bite plate worn after orthodontic treatment. A mold is made to your upper teeth for one half of the appliance, and your lower teeth for the other half. The device has additional hardware that keeps your lower jaw thrust out in front of your upper jaw. It is only worn while you sleep. It helps bring your tongue forward, so it does not slide backwards in your throat and block your airway. It can be a very effective way to treat mild sleep apnea. Some patients tolerate an oral appliance more easily than a CPAP device. Many dentists will fit you for this appliance, but only a small number in each city fully devote themselves to fitting these appliances for sleep apnea treatment.

Continuous Positive Airway Pressure, or CPAP, is basically a vacuum cleaner working in reverse. Instead of a motor generating suction to pull air into the machine, it blows out continuous air pressure to maintain the airway in your throat from collapsing. A mask needs to be worn over your nose and mouth, or in certain designs just your nose. As with many things, CPAP technology mask designs continue to improve. So, if your doctor tells you that you need CPAP, please give it a try. It could save your life.

CHAPTER TEN

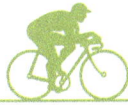

QUESTIONS OUR "KEEP HAMMERING IT" CLIENTS ASK

F or me, the Vail Method is a labor of love. I've devoted the past few years to getting the program and all its various elements just right. As part of that effort, I have drawn from all the resources at hand, everything from personal experiences to scholarly research. I have also tapped friends and colleagues who specialize in diet, exercise, sleep, meditation, and all the other fields that factor into the Vail Method. And I have walked the talk my entire adult life. Since college, I have been an avid long-distance runner and have often been teased for how healthy I eat and my decades-long aversion to fried foods and red meat. In med school I gulped fish oil and tested my cholesterol. I have tried various tests and assorted approaches to diet, running, and exercise. Of course, as with any project, some of those trials have resulted in errors. In the end, the brainstorming and experimentation have proved instrumental in creating a program I am certain will help many people lead healthier lives as they advance into their fifties and beyond.

But the method will only succeed if followed on a day-to-day, week-to-week basis. It must be a plan that you can embrace and make part of your everyday life. To help determine how well it works on a practical level, I sought feedback from friends and acquaintances who I thought might be intrigued about it or benefit from it. I described the Vail Method program to them. Everyone I queried was in the demographic I had in mind in devising the program: all were in their late forties and up; all had shown some interest in a healthy diet and exercise. I asked for their reactions, questions, thoughts, and concerns.

The responses—and in particular the questions—have been terrific. I suspect that many of you will have similar questions to those raised by my informal focus group. I decided to devote this chapter to some of the most interesting questions I received, along with my answers. I hope that this back and forth will inspire many of you to engage in a dialogue with me and other enthusiasts about the Vail Method.

Bob, a forty-nine-year-old consultant based in Florida, was a high school and college athlete who has attempted to keep up with an exercise routine. But with a busy business and family life, he cannot always squeeze a workout into his day. He is concerned about whether he is fit enough to take part in the rigorous training program outlined in the Vail Method. "What's the difference between level 101 and 201?" he asked. "How do I know if I qualify for 201?"

A major difference between a level 101 lifestyle person and 201 is a readiness to commit to training and to the other aspects of the program. People at the 201 level may not be in the best running or biking form of their life. But if they are reasonably fit and are willing to sign on to and stick with a regular exercise program, that qualifies them for a 201 level. In contrast, a 101 person will read books and magazine articles or seek advice, but only follow the program intermittently, for a shorter duration, and at a lower intensity than is needed to push the needle to a better place. Instead of walking briskly for an hour, they'll cut it to a twenty-minute stroll with the dog. The lower-intensity, shorter walk is not enough to make significant changes. Similar to New Year's resolution folks who join a gym in January and stop going by February, level 101 people frequently don't stay committed to a diet or an exercise program.

A 201-level person would ideally be exercising at least a couple of days a week for forty-five minutes or longer. And he or she should be actively seeking ways to improve fitness or prepare for a race.

Suzanne, a forty-five-year-old office manager and marathon runner in Chicago, was concerned that a plant-based diet was not something that she could stick with 100 percent of the time. "I've tried a vegetarian diet, and it just doesn't work for me," she said. "I lost too much weight. And I had cravings for fish and chicken. How strictly do you have to adhere to a vegetarian diet for the plan to work?"

We want you to understand the ideal diet, and then find your place or zone in it. The data and research points to a plant-based diet as the ideal. It has been shown to result in improved cardiovascular health, longevity, reduced diabetes, and lower risk for cancer.

In terms of craving animal meat, this is more usually related to seeing others eating foods that you are used to consuming, and battling mental cravings rather than physical. The aroma of certain foods can trigger emotions of comfort and happiness, memories of gatherings with family and friends. Part of the challenge of transitioning to a plant-based diet is overcoming the common concern that we are not getting enough protein.

If you eat small amounts of fish or dairy, it won't kill you. In fact, when we look at the Blue Zone—regions of the world where people live much longer than usual—we find that most inhabitants had small amounts of animal protein in their diet, so relax a little. Even in the Seventh Day Adventist population in Loma Linda, California, the vegetarians who ate some fish lived the longest.

The important thing is to find something that works for you. You need to find options for when you are eating out and socializing with friends and traveling. Restaurants are becoming more open toward creating meat-free options when asked. There are plenty of additional health benefits from the Vail Method, so don't get hung up on the vegetarian diet alone.

Part of how flexible you can be in your eating depends on your overall physical health and risk factors. If you are a healthy person with good cholesterol levels, low risk factors for heart disease, healthy body weight and body fat, and no insulin or blood sugar issues, you have more wiggle room in your nutrition. But understand that the more you adhere to the ideal diet, the healthier you will be. If you're overweight and diabetic or prediabetic, or have a family history of cardiovascular disease, it would be wise for you to closely follow a plant-based diet.

As you work on figuring out the best eating plan for you, here are some useful general principles to keep in mind:

- Learn not to fear carbohydrates. They should comprise most of your calories, and you need them to support healthy aerobic exercise.

- Remember that you don't need as much protein as you've been led to believe. In Blue Zone areas, where longevity is above average, protein consumption is quite low.

- Learn to talk less about "diets" (keto, gluten free, low carb, etc.) and more about nourishing your body with the proper amount of nutrients and calories to meet your needs. Continue to measure your weight, percent body fat, and glycogen stores for assessment of adequate nutrition.

Roger, a university professor in Washington, DC, asked how people who signed up for the Vail Method can track whether they are achieving their goals. "How will I know whether the Vail Method is working for me?" he asked. "What are the markers?"

It's a good question. Whenever we commit ourselves to something long term and demanding, we want to track what the payoff is. In the case of the Vail Method, there are some significant empirical ways to chart its effectiveness. One of them is weight loss. For those of us who put on several pounds once we hit middle age, being able to shed that spare tire is no small feat. In addition, you should see a decided drop in blood cholesterol and hemoglobin AIC levels, which reflect your average blood sugar over time. These tests will be part of your annual physical. Make sure that you ask your doctor for the results and keep records.

In your training, you should also find yourself able to run or bike more with the same amount of exertion and fatigue that shorter runs or rides have caused in the past. You should be wearing a heart monitor when you exercise and recording your training on a website diary or app on your phone. Watch and track what happens to your heart rate after you run or bike a couple of miles and how much more quickly you return to your resting heart rate when you complete your workout. With time, you will be training like an athlete, running at the zone 2 levels I discussed in chapter 6. Your pace will improve and your longer runs will become easier.

Sticking with the method will also increase the size and number of your mitochondria and your ability to clear lactate as you exercise. This enables you to increase your endurance and improve your performance. In chapter 6 I discuss how the lactate threshold test helps us evaluate your fitness. It's very rewarding to repeat the lactate test and see your improvement.

I also recommend that you participate in races—ideally the same races every year—and track your times. For those who don't have the time to train for a marathon or half marathon, five- and ten-kilometer races work just fine. As I mentioned in chapter 6, I take part in the Bolder Boulder 10K race every spring in Colorado. I have mostly managed to maintain or improve my time every year for the past five years, despite obviously getting older. If my pace has dropped in any given year, I picked it back up the following year. The race motivates me to compete with one person: me. This year I decided to mix in a half marathon, just to motivate myself, and build those endurance miles beyond my comfort zone of regular six- to seven-mile runs.

Finally, you should also pay attention to the subjective markers available to all of us. You should have increased energy to do more of everything, including work and exercise. You should also have a stronger sense of mindfulness and a feeling of being more at peace despite enduring the same craziness in your life.

Jack, a sixty-year-old restaurant owner in Baltimore, wonders how the Vail Method is better than the diet and exercise plan he's already using. "What can your plan do for me that would go beyond just keeping up a good exercise schedule and a healthy diet?" he asked.

As we've seen, the Vail Method is not just another diet and/or exercise book. It is a guide to healthy living backed by science and research. What is the good exercise schedule that you refer to? Are you monitoring your heart rate and do you know what it should be at in zone 2, for maximum improvement.? Also, what most people believe is a healthy diet is often far from it. The diet we promote is based on published scientific data in medical journals. The lifestyle in the Vail Method is the result of more than twenty-five years of experience with patients, and it includes the steps to minimize medical problems and allow for a vibrant, healthy life as we get older. It is the best answer to a lifelong frustration I often hear: "Dr. Ehrlich, there are no golden years." Yes, there can be. But like everything we've got to work for them.

Allison and Walter, a recently retired couple in their late fifties from Boston, think that the Vail Method might be just the thing that they need to jump-start their healthy living program as empty nesters. "We want to come to Vail and get initiated," they said. "How can we make that happen?"

Look for further information on our website **www.vailmethod.com.**

"I am pretty sold on the Vail Method," wrote Nick, a writer in Seattle. "My wife is skeptical. How can I convince her that it's good for both of us?"

We lead by example. When your wife sees you looking fitter and trimmer with more energy, she'll want "what he's having" as the famous line goes in *When Harry Met Sally*. Actually, the line is, "what she's having," but you get the point.

You should not expect to win her over in a day. Invite her on a hike, a run, or a bike ride with you. If your budget allows, take her on a group cycling tour like the one I described in chapter 4. She'll love you for it. Prepare a great plant-based meal for her. Take her out to a vegetarian restaurant. Bit by bit, she will likely appreciate sharing a lifestyle that you're enthusiastic about. The time together will be invaluable for couples who have split into one who is recreationally active and one who is not.

Also, be aware that she might never fully jump into the program. The Vail Method is so all-encompassing, it's good if our partners can be involved. But sometimes it does not work out that way. If your wife remains skeptical, it's not the end of the world. You're responsible for your destiny and health.

Greta, a teacher in Austin, Texas, is worried about selling a plant-based diet to her family. "I can see sticking to a vegetarian diet could work well for me," she said. "But my kids, who are teenagers, want to eat other things. How do I bring them on board?

This is a great question that addresses a common problem, a family divided by different dietary preferences or choices. For children and teenagers there are many recipes that mimic several of their favorite comfort foods such as vegan mac and cheese. With a little searching you'll find some that work for you.

In my household, the challenge is that I follow a plant-based diet, my wife is strictly meat and potatoes, and our teenagers are ... well, they're teenagers. One day they eat hamburgers and the next day they find meat repulsive. One day they'll eat spaghetti and tomato sauce and the next week, they say, "Mom, you know I don't like this."

One key is to make the change gradually. While you stick to your plant-based diet, you can start by occasionally serving a great vegetarian dish that the whole family can enjoy together. With time, they will likely realize that plant-based dishes can also be tasty.

Jack, a fifty-one-year-old entrepreneur from Denver, runs a couple of marathons a year. "I am pretty committed to a rigorous workout regime, running almost daily, etc.," he said. "How do I gauge if my body is overworked?"

If you are overtraining, you will begin to feel the signs. How much energy or spring do your legs have on runs or bike rides? Also, pay attention to your heart rate. If you are overtraining or not getting adequate rest and recovery you will notice that your heart rate does not rise to the level it normally does for a given degree of exertion. You will learn the heart rates that accompany your normal running pace(s) and will see that a hill or incline or pace that normally takes you to a certain level will not.

Be like the pros and take it easy when you need to. Switch to a resistance workout in the gym, or an easier run or bike ride.

Also, watch out for the culprits that contribute to overtraining. There is more to it than the amount of running or biking miles or sessions per week. Other factors are adequate nutrition—both total calories and carbohydrates appropriate for your amount of exercise and body weight. Many people trying to exercise as part of a weight-loss program will cut their carbohydrates, but as we discuss in detail in chapter 4, carbohydrates are the fuel for your engine. Also, look at how much sleep you are getting. Is it enough? Stress and lack of relaxation will also take their toll on you. Finally, if you are traveling frequently, you might need some time off or easier workouts to recover from large time zone changes.

Nancy is a single mother and small business owner based in St. Louis. Her worry is whether she can fit the program in as she juggles multiple demands on her time. "It seems like there are many aspects to the Vail Method program," she wrote. "I'm a busy person with many time pressures. For example, I don't always have time to meditate. How can I make this work for me?"

Time is the most precious thing in our busy lives. As with all things on our "to do" lists, we have to prioritize what we can and want to do. I find myself getting ready in the morning, doing my stretches, and shortening my meditation or replacing it with a minute or so of deep breathing and relaxation in order to get my run in before work, or make it to the office on time. The run has its own meditative or relaxing value to me, so that's an easy choice. When time allows, and I'm not pressured, I can take fifteen minutes to meditate when it will be more meaningful. This usual means another day or time. Our program is individualized to you. For some, weight management and health issues will be the most important areas, leading you to focus on the nutrition and exercise components. For others, sleep and mindfulness take center stage. There is something for everyone to benefit from in this program.

Roger is a media executive in Atlanta. "Can I expect that engaging in the Vail Method will enhance my sex drive?" he asked. "Are regular testosterone shots a necessity for a heightened sex drive?"

The human sex drive is a complicated biological process involving physical and emotional factors. As you advance in the Vail Method you will see an improvement in body weight and lean muscle mass. This should improve your self-image. In turn, this may improve your interest in sex (or your partner's). Another part of the program is monitoring your sex hormones and treating low levels. Low testosterone will decrease your sex drive, and restoration to healthy physiologic levels will help. If you are one of the fortunate ones who has good testosterone levels, there is no reason to boost them higher with testosterone shots. Also, do not confuse sex drive with sexual performance. Erectile dysfunction (ED), discussed in chapter 3, is a vascular, or atherosclerotic hardening of the arteries problem. A plant-based diet has anecdotally helped some ED patients with improved circulation and performance.

Sam, a fifty-six-year-old New Yorker, noted that we encourage everyone to take several tests when they start the Vail Method. "Are the lactate threshold test and the other tests you recommend something I should do once and be done with them?" he asked. "Or should they become part of my regular physical checkups?"

The lactate threshold test is done at a sports medicine center or other medical facility and not during a yearly family doctor's physical. It does make sense to repeat the test as you make progress in your fitness. The target heart rate that you train at in zone 2 may well be different as you improve your fitness. Also, if you are active in both running and biking, ideally you would be tested separately in each modality, on the treadmill, and on a special bike in the lab. However, most recreational athletes would not be tested yearly on a regular basis.

Eddie, fifty-five, based in Asheville, North Carolina, is a lifelong runner. But he is considering shifting over to mostly biking. "Some other specialists have said that running is not good for the knees and other joints as we get older," he said. "They recommend that we shift more to cycling and other forms of physical exercise. And yet, you seem to encourage running as part of the Vail Method. What's your position on that?"

Running is actually helpful for the joints. The mechanism is not completely understood, but somehow the impact of running helps lubricate the joints and preserve the cartilage. The challenge is to maintain strength in our core, gluteals, and hips, and to deal with imbalances that are causing problems and pain. That's why a good fitness program should include regular stretching and core exercises. I described a good balanced approach you can take in chapter 6. But if your joints are healthy, continued running will not hurt you, and is actually beneficial. Road biking is great though too; mixing them up is even better.

Julie, a forty-nine-year-old homemaker in Illinois, was not sure about our approach to supplements. "I note that you are somewhat skeptical about supplements," she wrote. "But, as a woman, I have found that taking supplements on a regular basis helps me maintain hormonal balance. So, can I expect to need them less as I get more engaged with the Vail Method?"

Hormonal replacement through bio identical hormones or use of herbal supplements is an important part of managing the aging process. The Vail Method will not replace the need for them. If some supplements work for you, by all means keep using them.

In terms of other supplements, think of healthy food as medicine for your body and soul. By making sure you are getting adequate calories and nutrients to maintain your energy, weight, and muscle mass, you will achieve the greatest benefit to your health. In the lab, we enjoy seeing people return to repeat their lactate threshold tests and perform better just by putting them on an appropriate diet!

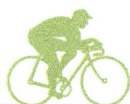

FINAL THOUGHTS

T hanks for reading this far. One more page and you will reach the finish line! I am grateful that you have made the time to take in what the Vail Method is about.

Now I want to know: Did it inspire you? Are you motivated? Ready to sign on?

I mean you, the one who is trying to figure out how to trim down your marathon time.

And you, whose brain is constantly dashing between mental to-do lists—work duties, home chores, and family responsibilities—and are looking for a way to calm the whirring in your mind. And you, too, the one who has tried more weight-loss diets than you can count and just want a solid reliable plan for healthy eating.

What I have outlined in these pages is the best way I know to get you—all of you—out of your ruts and into healthier, more active and productive lives. And to protect your health for the long run! Whether your search is for a better workout plan, diet guidance, or improved mindfulness—or all three, and more—this book was designed with you in mind. It's about fine-tuning your good exercise and eating habits, throwing out the bad ones, and creating new and better ones. The overarching goal is putting you solidly on that 201 level of exercise and living, and preventing the chronic diseases that plague the Western world.

By this point you know the Vail Method encompasses more than exercise and healthier eating. It's a blueprint for a better lifestyle. Each of the elements I have detailed in these pages is a crucial component of that lifestyle. Unless you cheated and skipped some pages, you're familiar with the various components: (1) a diet centered around whole plant foods, (2) an aerobic exercise program guided by your optimum heart rate scientifically determined by your lactate levels, (3) a physical therapy plan tailored to your musculoskeletal imbalances and weaknesses to keep you moving, (4) sound rest and sleep habits, and (5) a way to still your mind on a regular basis.

If all that seems like a lot to bite off at once, I recommend going at it in small increments. Run a little harder. Eat more veggies. Meditate with more concentration. Step by step, you will get there and we will keep you there.

At the same time, this lifestyle is the key to avoiding heart disease, diabetes, and other chronic ailments that reduce our quality of life. Not only will you feel better and stronger, lose weight, and be happier with exercise, a plant-based diet, and mindfulness, but your future health will be brighter too.

So, let's get up and get started! And to continue the conversation, visit us at **www.drmattehrlich.com**, or **www.vailmethod.com**.

ENDNOTES

1 Frederico G. S. Toledo, Simon Watkins, and David E. Kelley, "Changes Induced by Physical Activity and Weight Loss in the Morphology of Intermyofibrillar Mitochondria in Obese Men and Women," *Journal of Clinical Endocrinology & Metabolism* 9, no. 8 (August 2006): 3224-2337, https://doi.org/10.1210/jc.2006-0002.;

2 J. Hill and I. San Millan, "Validation of Musculoskeletal Ultrasound to Assess and Quantify Muscle Glycogen Content. A Novel Approach," *The Physician and Sportsmedicine* 42, no. 3 (Sept. 2014), 45-52, https://doi.org/10.3810/psm.2014.09.2075.

3 A. Draeger, "Statin Therapy Induces Ultrastructural Damage in Skeletal Muscle in Patients without Myalgia," *Journal of Pathology* 210, no. 1 (Sept. 2006): 94-102, https://doi.org/10.1002/path.2018.

4 Markus G. Mohaupt et al., "Association between Statin-Associated Myopathy and Skeletal Muscle Damage," *CMAJ* 181, no. 1-2 (July 7, 2009): E11-E18, DOI: https://doi.org/10.1503/cmaj.081785.

5 Thomas Colin Campbell, "A Plant-Based Diet and Animal Protein: Questioning Dietary Fat and Considering Animal Protein As the Main Cause of Heart Disease," Journal of Geriatric Cardiology 14, no. 5 (May 2017): 331-337, doi: 10.11909/j.issn.1671-5411.2017.05.011;

R. S. Najjar, C. E. Moore, and B. D. Montgomery, "A Defined, Plant-Based Diet Utilized in an Outpatient Cardiovascular Clinic Effectively Treats Hypercholesterolemia and Hypertension and Reduces Medications," Clinical Cardiology 41, no. 3 (March 2018): 307-313, doi: 10.1002/clc.22863;

D. Ornish et al., "Effects of Stress Management Training and Dietary Changes in Treating Ischemic Heart Disease," JAMA

249, no. 1 (January 1983): 54-59, https://www.ncbi.nlm.nih.gov/pubmed/6336794;

D. Ornish et al., "Can Lifestyle Changes Reverse Coronary Heart Disease? The Lifestyle Heart Trial," Lancet 336, no. 8717 (September 22, 1990): 129-133, https://www.thelancet.com/journals/lancet/article/PII0140-6736(90)91656-U/fulltext;

C. B. Esselstyn Jr., "Updating a 12-year Experience with Arrest and Reversal Therapy for Coronary Heart Disease (an Overdue Requiem for Palliative Cardiology)," American Journal of Cardiology 84, no. 3 (August 1991): 339-341, https://www.ajconline.org/article/S0002-9149(99)00290-8/fulltext.

6 Abou Kane-Diallo et al., "Association between a Pro Plant-Based Dietary Score and Cancer Risk in the Prospective NutriNet-Santé Cohort," International Journal of Cancer 142, no. 10 (May 2018), https://doi.org/10.1002/ijc.31593;

World Cancer Research Fund/American Institute for Cancer Research, "Food, Nutrition, Physical Activity, and the Prevention of Cancer: A Global Perspective," 2007.

7 Mingyang Song et al., "Association of Animal and Plant Protein Intake with All-Cause and Cause-Specific Mortality," JAMA Internal Medicine 176, no. 10 (October 2016): 1453–1463, doi: 10.1001/jamainternmed.2016.4182;

Michael J. Orlich et al., "Vegetarian Diet Patterns and Mortality in Adventist Health Study 2," JAMA Internal Medicine 173, no. 13 (July 2013): 1230-1238, doi: 10.1001/jamainternmed.2013.6473.

8 Zhangling Chen et al., "Plant Versus Animal Based Diets and Insulin Resistance, Prediabetes and Type 2 Diabetes: the Rotterdam Study," European Journal of Epidemiology 33, No. 9 (September

2018): 883-893, https://doi.org/10.1007/s10654-018-0414-8(0123456789().,-volV)(0123456789().,-volV);

S. Tonstad et al., "Vegetarian Diets and Incidence of Diabetes in the Adventist Health Study-2," *Nutrition, Metabolism & Cardiovascular Diseases* 23, no. 4 (April 2013): 292-299, https://doi.org/10.1016/j.numecd.2011.07.004.

9 Najjar et al., op. cit.

10 X. Gao et al., "Prospective Study of Dietary Pattern and Risk of Parkinson Disease," *American Journal of Clinical Nutrition* 86, no. 5 (November 2007): 1486-1494, doi: 10.1093/ajcn/86.5.1486;

S. P. Shah and J. E. Duda, "Dietary Modifications in Parkinson's Disease: A Neuroprotective Intervention?" *Medical Hypotheses* 85, no. 6 (December 2015): doi: 10.1016/j.mehy.2015.08.018.

11 Campbell, op. cit.

12 Ornish et al., op. cit.

13 Fiona S. Atkinson, Kaye Foster-Powell, and Jennie C. Brand-Miller, "International Tables of Glycemic Index and Glycemic Load Values: 2008," *Diabetes Care* 31, no. 12 (December 2008): 2281-2283, doi: 10.2337/dc08-1239.

14 Samantha Solon-Biet et al., "Macronutrients and Caloric Intake in Health and Longevity," *Journal of Endocrinology,* 226, no. 1 (July 2015): R17–R28, doi: 10.1530/JOE-15-0173;

Valter Longo, *The Longevity Diet: Discover the New Science Behind Stem Cell Activation and Regeneration to Slow Aging, Fight Disease, and Optimize Weight* (New York: Avery, 2018).

15 Nicole Brady, "Tests Find Potential Toxins in Popular Protein Powders," The Denver Channel, May 26, 2018, https://

www.thedenverchannel.com/news/local-news-tests-find-poten-
tial-toxins-in-popular-protein-powders.

16 S. Potgieter, "Sports Nutrition: A Review of the Latest
Guidelines for Exercise and Sports Nutrition from the American
College of Sport Nutrition, the International Olympic Committee,
and the International Society for Sports Nutrition," *South African
Journal of Clinical Nutrition* 26, no. 1 (January 2013): 6-16, http://
sajcn.co.za/index.php/SAJCN/article/view/685.

17 Ibid.

18 Ibid.

19 C. Kersick et. al., "International Society of Sports Nutrition
Position Stand: Nutrient Timing," *Journal of the International Society
of Sports Nutrition* 14, no. 33 (July 2017), https://jissn.biomedcen-
tral.com/articles/10.1186/s12970-017-0189-4.

20 Potgieter, op. cit.

21 Ibid.

22 R. Jager et al., "International Society of Sports Nutrition
Position Stand: Protein and Exercise," *Journal of the International
Society of Sports Nutrition* 14, no. 20 (June 2017);

M. Mazzulla et al., "Endurance Exercise Attenuates Postprandial
Whole-Body Leucine Balance in Trained Men," *Medicine & Science
in Sports & Exercise* 49, no. 12 (December 2017): 2585-2592, doi:
10.1249/MSS.0000000000001394.

23 A. E. Harper, "Evolution of Recommended Dietary Allow-
ances—New Directions?" *Annual Review of Nutrition* 7 (1987):
509-537; G. Davis, *Proteinaholic: How Our Obsession with Meat Is*

Killing Us and What We Can Do About It (New York: Harper Collins, 2015).

24 Potgieter, op. cit.

25 Ibid.

26 Orlich et al., op. cit.

27 D. Buettner, *The Blue Zones Solution: Eating and Living Like the World's Healthiest People* (Washington, DC: National Geographic Partners, 2015).

28 Ibid.

29 D. Ornish et al., "Intensive Lifestyle Changes May Affect the Progression of Prostate Cancer," *Journal of Urology* 174, no. 3 (Sept. 2005): 1065-1069, doi: 10.1097/01.ju.0000169487.49018.73.

30 Dean Ornish, "An Update on the Evidence Behind Lifestyle Medicine" (lecture, Advances in Cardiovascular Disease Prevention Understanding the Latest in Medications, Lifestyle, and Risk Factor Reduction, Saint Joseph Hospital, Denver, CO, October 12, 2018).

31 K. Maruyama et al., "Exposure to Exogenous Estrogen Through Intake of Commercial Milk from Pregnant Cows," *Pediatrics International* 52, no. 1 (February 2010): 33-8.

32 A. Dagfinn et al., "Dairy Products, Calcium, and Prostate Cancer Risk: A Systematic Review and Meta-Analysis of Cohort Studies," *American Journal of Clinical Nutrition* 101, no. 1 (January 2015): 87–117, https://doi.org/10.3945/ajcn.113.067157;

W. Lu et al., "Dairy Products Intake and Cancer Mortality Risk: A Meta-Analysis of 11 Population Based Cohort Studies," *American Journal of Clinical Nutrition* 101, no. 1 (January 2015): 87–117, https://doi.org/10.3945/ajcn.113.067157.

33　K. Hughes et al., "Intake of Dairy Foods and Risk of Parkinson Disease," Neurology 89, no. 1 (July 4, 2017): 46–52, doi: [10.1212/WNL.0000000000004057];

W. Jiang et al., "Dairy Foods Intake and Risk of Parkinson's Disease: A Dose-Response Meta-Analysis of Prospective Cohort Studies," *European Journal of Epidemiology* 29, no. 9 (September 2014): 613-619, https://doi.org/10.1007/s10654-014-9921-4.

34 J.　Dua et al., "Residue Behavior of Organochlorine Pesticides During the Production Process of Yogurt and Cheese," *Food Chemistry* 15, no. 245 (October 2017): 119-124. doi: 10.1016/j. foodchem.2017.10.017.

35　Hughes et al., op. cit.

36　W. Han et al., "Scale and Causes of Lead Contamination in Chinese Tea," *Environmental Pollution* 139, no. 1 (January 2006): 125-32. Epub 2005 Jul 5, DOI: 10.1016/j.envpol.2005.04.025;

C. Peng et al., "Aluminum and Heavy Metal Accumulation in Tea Leaves: An Interplay of Environmental and Plant Factors and an Assessment of Exposure Risks to Consumers," *Journal of Food Science* 83, no. 4 (April 2018): 1165-1172. doi: 10.1111/1750-3841.14093. Epub 2018 Mar 25.

37　Patrick J. Gray et al., "Cooking Rice in Excess Water Reduces Both Arsenic and Enriched Vitamins in the Cooked Grain," *Food Additives & Contaminants* 33, no. 1 (October 2015): 78-85, DOI: 10.1080/19440049.2015.1103906;

D. Wilson, "Arsenic Consumption in the United States," *Journal of Environmental Health* 78, no. 3 (October 2015): 8-14.

38　Gray et al., op. cit.

39 C. Kerksick et al., "ISSN Exercise & Sports Nutrition Review Update: Research and Recommendations," *Journal of the International Society of Sports Nutrition* 15, no. 38 (August 2018), https://jissn.biomedcentral.com/articles/10.1186/s12970-018-0242-y.

40 Ibid.

41 Ibid.

42 E. Rawson et al., "Dietary Supplements for Health, Adaptation, and Recovery in Athletes," *International Journal of Sport Nutrition and Exercise Metabolism* 28, no. 2 (March 2018): 188-199, https://doi.org/10.1123/ijsnem.2017-0340.

43 M. Sellami et al., "Herbal Medicine for Sports: A Review," *Journal of the International Society of Sports Nutrition* 15, no. 14 (March 2018), https://doi.org/10.1186/s12970-018-0218-y.

44 Mona Ghasemian, Sina Owlia, and Mohammad Bagher Owlia, "Review of Anti-Inflammatory Herbal Medicines," *Advances in Pharmacological Sciences* 2016, Article ID 9130979 (2016), http://dx.doi.org/10.1155/2016/9130979.

45 Christiane Northrup, *The Wisdom of Menopause* (New York: Bantam Dell, 2006), 181-187;

Sara Gottfried, *The Hormone Cure: Reclaim Balance, Sleep, Sex Drive & Vitality Naturally with the Gottfried Protocol* (New York: Scribner, 2013), 109-113.

46 F. Watanabe, "Vitamin B12-Containing Plant Food Sources for Vegetarians," *Nutrients* 6, no. 5 (May 2014): 1861-1873, doi:10.3390/nu6051861.

47 R. T. Ras, J. M. Geleijnse, and E. I. Trautwein, "LDL-Cholesterol-Lowering Effect of Plant Sterols and Stanols Across Different

Dose Ranges: A Meta-Analysis of Randomised Controlled Studies," *British Journal of Nutrition* 112, no. 2 (July 2014): 214–219, doi: 10.1017/S0007114514000750.

48 M. C. Pascoe, D. R. Thompson, and C. F. Ski, "Yoga, Mindfulness-Based Stress Reduction and Stress-Related Physiological Measures: A Meta-Analysis," *Psychoneuroendocrinology* 86 (December 2017): 152-168, doi: 10.1016/j.psyneuen.2017.08.008.

Printed in the USA
CPSIA information can be obtained
at www.ICGtesting.com
LVHW071205101123
763485LV00101B/4353

9 781949 639506